To Cindy + Bob,

Thank you
and God Bless You,

Jamie Renee Thomas

Cancer-Free

Naturally

A New Approach

to

Outsmarting Cancer

RENEE THOMAS

Terminal Breast Cancer Survivor

ISBN: 9781690765844

FRM Publishing
6801 Brookeshire Dr. Suite 101
West Bloomfield, Michigan 48322
Email: Faye@frmpublishing.com
Website: FRMpublishing.com

Printed in the U.S.A

Foreword

There are more ways to eliminate cancer from our bodies than modern medicine offers us. I have been in complete remission from terminal breast cancer for nearly four years. According to my oncologist, it's pretty extraordinary to be in full remission for so long. The reaction I get when I tell people about it is, "Wow, that's amazing", or "That's incredible" and most importantly to them, "What did you do?" I have gladly shared this information with anyone who asked for it. I cannot promise that these methods will work for you, but I believe that if you have cancer, you will get better and possibly live longer than you otherwise would if you become your own doctor like I did.

I am sure if I had relied on mainstream medicine alone, I would probably be dead by now. They as much as told me so. My medical team helped me to live with cancer, but they couldn't cure it. They did many wonderful things for me but basically expected me to die. I think the main reason I survived this long is because I believed I would. My belief in a Higher Power led me to search and find alternative methods that could cure the cancer that was invading my body. Because of that faith, I am cancer-free. Everything I used to get healthy again is included in this book. I made many changes, so I can't be sure if any one treatment or supplement is individually responsible for my recovery.

Nearly all of the information found between these pages is available from multiple sources online or in magazines or books. I have tried to give credit to each source, but when I was searching for help, I often scribbled down information quickly and moved on. At that time, I had no intention of writing a book on being cured because I was supposed to succumb to the disease before 2016. If you are a cancer victim, please feel free to use my experience and resources as part of your own research. I have included as much information as I can about how I lived through the roughest time in my life. This is my journal on how I overcame terminal breast cancer. I can't be sure, but it may be possible that these methods work on other types of cancer as well. Since I am not a medical professional, I cannot give you medical advice on how you can cure your cancer. But I can share with you how I cured mine.

Acknowledgements

I wish to acknowledge my brother Tom whose research gave me the most valuable step in my recovery, and whose persistence gave me the courage to try it.

I am also grateful to my editor Faye Menczer Ascher whose expertise and assistance made this book possible.

DEDICATION

I will never forget the beloved members of my family whose lives were taken by cancer. Their suffering inspired me to find real hope for cancer victims and to share it with the world.

To my sons Jeff and James, who make my life brighter and give me a reason to want to keep on living.

TABLE of CONTENTS

1: Cancer Takes up Residence in my Body   6

2: Why is Cancer so Puzzling?   31

3: Going "Au Naturel"   39

4: I Believe I can Survive   45

5: Why I Don't Believe in Chemotherapy   51

6: From Cancer Patient to Cancer Survivor   58

7: What is the Cost of a Pound of Sugar?   67

8: Toss Your Junk and Get the Lead Out   74

9: It's Never Too Late   80

10: A Skin Cream That Can Heal Cancer?   87

11: Vitamins and Minerals to Take for Life   96

12: Life Goes On   114

References   119

Chapter 1:
Cancer Takes up Residence
in My Body

By most standards, I am a typical American woman. I have a college degree, worked as a Social Worker for the majority of my life. I've been married and divorced. I raised two wonderful boys as a mostly single parent. I do not have any special training in cancer research. Let me assure you I am no genius. I do not even have a medical background. I skipped nursing school because during my senior year in high school I went to visit a friend who was hospitalized after being injured in a motorcycle accident. He had skinned his arm raw from elbow to wrist, and while I was visiting him, a nurse came in to change his bandages. When I saw his unwrapped arm all pink and red with what looked like dirt still embedded in it, I rushed from his room to a hallway bathroom and dry heaved. Then I left with a change of heart about a nursing career. I have always become weak in the knees when someone talks about their physical pains or past surgeries. I had no interest in the medical field, unless I was sick or injured. During my lifetime I had acquired a healthy skepticism of pharmaceutical drugs. I believe most medical doctors and researchers are good people, and much smarter than I am. Because I am far from wealthy, I could never afford the latest and greatest cutting edge cancer treatment that costs thousands a month. I am both a victim of cancer and an observer of its toll on others. Since the 1980's, even with the best medical intervention, I have seen people fall ill and die from it, including friends, family members, and clients on my caseload. It seems very little has changed over the years. Statistically, nearly everyone has a friend or family member who is struggling with cancer or has died from it. Cancer is a fearsome invader. It does not discriminate by age, gender, or how much money you make. It strikes rich and poor. It has a very successful history of killing most of its victims in spite of billions of dollars and years of research devoted to it. Nearly half of all men and women in America will be diagnosed with cancer sometime in their lives. One in eight women will be diagnosed with breast cancer during her life. According to Cancer.org, almost two million new cases of cancer are diagnosed each year, and over six hundred thousand die from it annually. These are horrible statistics, and I became one of them.

The beginning of my cancer journey was very typical. Shortly after my 61st birthday in April of 2013, I felt a small lump in my left breast. It was so small, I wasn't sure it was anything to worry about, and I let it go. I considered myself pretty healthy for my age, although I was overweight at 175 pounds. After three months, it was still there. A mammogram revealed something suspicious, and I was referred to an oncologist. The first oncologist I consulted for a diagnosis before my lumpectomies in 2013 was a male doctor in his 60's that I'll call Dr. B. He recommended a biopsy and if positive, a lumpectomy and follow-up radiation of my left breast. The biopsy was positive for a very small spot. I was queasy about the idea of radiation, so he scheduled a pre-op consult with the radiologist to allay my fears. There, I learned that radiation of my left breast would "clip" my lung but not my heart, allegedly. It would theoretically kill any remaining cancer cells in my left breast but could possibly damage my left lung. I felt sure my heart or some important blood vessels would be in the line of fire. I was afraid of potential damage and I expressed concerns about the radiation causing lung cancer or heart damage. The radiologist replied that "it will be years before that happened" and I shouldn't worry about it. I got the impression he thought I would be dead before it could cause a secondary cancer, but I thought it just might bring about my future demise, so I declined his services.

During the second office visit with Dr. B., I told him I was not going to have radiation on my left breast. He was not pleased with my refusal and insisted I needed to follow his protocol of surgery, radiation and maybe chemo. During the course of the visit, I asked him about things that could have caused my breast cancer. To my surprise, he sidestepped the question. I asked if he thought aluminum in deodorants could be a factor, and he actually laughed as he told me there's no connection. So, I asked him again, "What does cause it then?" His answer: "We don't know." What? For someone who makes cancer treatment his career he had just admitted he had no answers as to why people get it. I almost wanted to scream at him, "Shouldn't you be doing some research into causes, so you can counsel your patients?" My next thought was: If you say you don't know what causes it, then how can you be so sure aluminum in deodorant isn't to blame when research shows a potential link?

The irony of his statements seemed completely

lost on him. He didn't know what causes cancer but knew for sure it wasn't aluminum in deodorants. It wasn't a trick question I just made up. I had done some preliminary research in between appointments that indicated aluminum stops sweating by plugging sweat glands in your armpits. It keeps you from perspiring, but aluminum is also absorbed through your skin and can migrate as a result of small nicks from shaving. I don't know for sure if there is a connection, but I'm not willing to risk it. I never went back to him. The biopsy had discovered a malignancy, but small and still at Stage 1. The diagnosis read:

> Left breast mass, infiltrating ductal carcinoma.
> ER: Positive (Estrogen receptors present; estrogen encourages cancer growth)
> PR: Negative, (Progesterone receptors not present, does not encourage cancer growth)
> HER-2 neu: Equivocal (+2) (can't be diagnosed as positive or negative)

I looked up what it means to have HER-2. Here's what I found from cancer.org: "HER-2 is a growth-promoting protein on the outside of all breast cells. If positive, these cancers tend to grow and spread faster than other breast cancers." With a diagnosis of HER 2 neutral or equivocal, it's unclear if it is positive or negative. I might have the faster growing cancer, or I might not. I optimistically assumed mine was the "not positive" kind of HER 2.

I found a wonderful female oncologist who seemed more receptive to my rebelliousness. I told her I did not want to do radiation or chemo and she was fine with that. I had delayed taking any action for about six months after I first felt a lump. It was a bad decision. Finally, on November 1st, I was scheduled for a lumpectomy and removal of the four closest lymph nodes leading to my left armpit, called sentinel nodes, to see if it had spread from the primary site on the side of my left breast. To my relief, my lymph nodes were clear, and I considered myself out of danger. But eleven days after the lumpectomy, I went back under anesthesia to get more breast tissue removed. The first surgery results revealed that there were still cancerous cells present along the edges of the removed tissue, and my cancer diagnosis was changed to Stage ll. I want to note that the reason for the delayed lab results was because the local hospital did not have the ability to test the specimen during the surgery. The sample had to be sent out to a lab in Columbus, Ohio, over a hundred miles away. If the lab could have tested the samples on-site, I would not have needed two separate surgeries. That may or may not be important in what happened later. The lab test following my second lumpectomy showed clear margins, meaning no signs of cancer cells lingered in my breast. Breast cancer cells can travel away from the initial site and show up months or years later in soft tissue, organs, and in bones. When it travels and starts to create tumors in multiple areas like bones or organs, it becomes known as Stage IV breast cancer. I didn't feel pressured to do anything more because the cancer had not invaded those first four lymph nodes. Radiation can bring its own risk of developing cancer later on, and its effectiveness is questionable.

Chemotherapy, from my observation, is a draconian measure that can hurtle a person faster toward death and cause great pain and mental agony along the way. I refused the anti-hormone pill

Letrozole also due to potential side effects. I decided to do the recommended regular oncology checkups even though I felt I was cured after the two lumpectomies. I made appointments with my doctor every six months.

For a year and a half, between the end of 2013 and the middle of 2015, everything was fine. I was cancer free, or so I thought. That meant I made no changes to my diet, which consisted of steaks, hamburgers, hot dogs, lunch meat, prepared box meals, sugary cereals and desserts and very few fruits or vegetables. I had discontinued the antiperspirant that had aluminum as a primary ingredient and that was about the only change I made. Luckily, the cancer never came back to my chest or breast area even though I was still fifty pounds overweight. I continued taking an herb called black cohosh, which I had been using since I underwent menopause at the age of fifty nine, two years prior to my cancer diagnosis. It seemed to help reduce hot flashes. I do not know if my continued use of this herb is in any way related to the return of the cancer, but it is said to mimic estrogen in the body. My type of breast cancer was estrogen sensitive. I put myself at risk for it to return because of what I did and didn't do.

I should not have waited for six months after I first suspected I had breast cancer. During that time, it went from Stage I to Stage II. Fear and denial had kept me from acting sooner. Once again, fear and denial kept me from believing it would come back.

In April 2015, two years to the month after my initial cancer symptoms, I lost the ability to walk or sleep on my left side. I was in constant pain in my hip, left leg, and lower back. I dragged my leg and winced getting in and out of my car. I chalked it up to arthritis from an old auto accident injury, for which I had been treated periodically by a chiropractor. So, I made an appointment with him. The X-ray he took of my hip and spine missed the almost transparent hole in my hip bone because the X-ray he took didn't reach high enough on my hip. After a full month of excruciating chiropractic adjustments on my hip and spine, I told him it wasn't helping and asked for a referral to someone else. He suggested I see an orthopedic physician, and I made an appointment at a local orthopedic clinic. There, I underwent an X-ray and CT scan of my left side and spine that showed a thinned area of bone on my hip. I was told to report to the local hospital the next day for an emergency total hip replacement. A fracture and the thinned areas of my hip were so large the doctor feared it would break just from turning over in bed.

So, the last Friday in May, just before Labor Day weekend, I was admitted to the hospital, and had an emergency titanium hip replacement done that afternoon. I didn't know why this had happened to me and the doctors said they needed to run tests to be sure of a diagnosis.

My hospital stay lasted eight days. After the first four days in the hospital, I started therapy to stand and walk with a walker. The pain was almost unbearable. Fortunately, I was sedated much of the time. When I experienced heart palpitations and an irregular heartbeat on the fifth day, I was transferred to the cardiac unit where I remained the other three days. I was diagnosed with an underlying heart condition, known as atrial fibrillation. Unchecked, it could lead to a heart attack or stroke. I had had heart palpitations for years prior to this time but kept it under control by taking CoQ10 and B vitamins and aspirin. At the hospital I didn't have access to them. So, the palpitations came back. I needed every one of those eight hospital days, because I was in severe pain and unable to walk more than a few steps even with a walker. While I was in the hospital, multiple tests were conducted including bone scans, X-rays, blood tests, CT scans, and others I can't remember because of the pain meds and the twilight haze I was in.

The tests revealed that I had no cancer cells in either breast, but breast cancer cells had migrated to my left hip. I got that news the day before I was discharged from a doctor I didn't recognize. He said he had seen me several times during my hospital stay, but I didn't remember him. You know how they usually come and stand right beside your bed? And maybe pat your hand? Not this one. He stood at the foot of my bed with his arms folded together. I knew then it was bad news. Like an arrow, his words pierced my foggy brain. "I am sorry to tell you that your hip fracture was caused by breast cancer cells that traveled to your bones. You have Stage IV Breast Cancer. It's still in your upper left femur, your spine, and possibly your skull, kidney and liver. We can't cure it."

What? I had Stage IV Breast Cancer? The diagnosis doesn't get any worse than that. He told me in a matter of fact way, but his eyes betrayed the pity he must have felt for me. I could only stare at him in disbelief and tell myself that it can't be true. "I'm not going to die from this, not now," I told myself. "I still have things I need to do." Yet the sadness in his eyes told me what my mind refused to believe. He had just given me a terminal diagnosis. When I asked about how much time I had, he said "possibly six months." In near panic, I asked him, "What am I supposed to do?" His parting words to me were, "Go home and enjoy the time you have left." Then he walked out of the room, leaving me alone to digest the death sentence he had just delivered.

I was too stunned to cry. I knew what it meant. A few months filled with ever increasing pain, because the cancer in my bones was very painful. I could not believe what he had said to me. It was like being an actor in a bad movie. It wasn't real, just a story line. Why was he lying to me like that? Why was he hurting me with his crazy words? I was in utter disbelief. What are people supposed to do when a doctor has just promised you death instead of a cure? I had the hip surgery. I should be healed. I had been lulled into a sense of security after my lumpectomy surgeries to remove cancer from my left breast when it was only Stage II. The only medical options I was given after this latest surgery was radiation and chemotherapy.

Everything was supposed to be good. My thoughts turned and twisted and grew morbid. I looked back at what had led up to this horrible outcome. I was first diagnosed in 2013 with Stage II breast cancer. It was gone I was told. Less than two years later, it progressed to Stage IV. Now, at age 63, breast cancer cells had metastasized to my bones and possibly my organs. I was told I was going to die before my next birthday. I was so confused about how this had happened I didn't know what to think. I got very depressed. I couldn't decide what to do. Should I just give up? Make my funeral arrangements? Get my papers in order? Go home and lie on the couch and wait for death? That's the decision I faced that awful morning in June of 2015.

I had a son at home who had three more years of college. How would he fare without me? I knew for his sake I had to live.

The day after receiving that terrible terminal diagnosis, I was given follow-up appointments to see my oncologist and a radiologist and discharged to a nursing home for intensive physical therapy. Because I could not walk more than a few steps and only with excruciating pain, the doctor talked me into going there and I agreed to go for a week. I went by ambulance to a nursing home close to my home that doubled as a rehab center. I was settled into a room with an elderly, mostly deaf woman who fortunately was ambulatory. I was told I could not get out of bed to use the bathroom, even though I knew I was able, until I was evaluated by their therapist the next day. By nine pm, I called a cab to take me home because it was an awful experience for many reasons. I was in a room with a woman who kept her TV on the loudest possible setting, so sleep would have been impossible. But mostly I felt I was just dumped there. Earlier that evening I used the call button for assistance to use the bathroom and they brought me a bed pan. A few minutes later, I used the call button, but no one came. After ten minutes more, my roommate went to the nursing station for me, but still no one came. Finally, I used my cell phone to call the nursing home front desk. Then someone came. The next call I made was for a ride home. When the taxi arrived, I was told I could not leave. Since I knew my rights, I told them I could. Losing the argument, they left my room and came back with a form I signed that said I was leaving AMA- against medical advice. No one on the staff came back in to help me gather my bags. One of them watched me from the nursing station as I walked with a walker to the front door, dragging my left leg behind me. I got home and flopped on my couch, unable to tackle even the stairs to my bedroom.

The next morning, I began to sort out what I could and couldn't do. I couldn't go back to work, because I couldn't drive, or even get in or out of a car without significant pain. So, money was going to be tight. I had no savings to speak of and I worried I was going to lose my home. I decided I could use my time and the internet to look up information on my disease and what other options there might be for me to try.

Fortunately, I didn't have to worry about the medical bills because of my state's "Breast and Cervical Cancer Project" program, (BCCP) which gives Medicaid coverage to eligible cancer victims. I found out about it just before my breast cancer diagnosis, when I had a mammogram done at the county public health women's clinic. There they gave me a brochure on the program. No other health professional had mentioned that I might qualify for it.

The reality was I had a terminal disease, but I also had a choice; to either accept death as inevitable or fight for my life. I chose to fight. I just felt that I didn't need to accept dying by Christmas. Cancer was the enemy I had to vanquish. Somehow, I would find a way to make that happen. I prayed, but I knew it would take more than prayer. I've always believed it helps in any challenge. I did expect to find the answer if I just did the work. I would be relentless until I conquered it, I decided. I spoke to God and prayed like I did when I was a little girl. Childhood memories came flooding back to me. Many times, while I attended Catholic grade school, and when I felt afraid, I would sneak into the empty church next door after school and kneel before the statue of the Virgin Mary and pray. I talked to her about my problems like she was a real mother figure. Once I looked up and saw her sad down-turned lips change briefly into a smile. It was an ecstatic moment that made me feel she heard me and sent her love. Now I prayed to her again, in my hour of need. The bible says that Jesus healed the sick, and made Lazarus come alive again. Jesus preached that faith in God the Father can move mountains. Maybe I could get a miracle too. I prayed for more time at least until my youngest son was able to fend for himself. I believe I heard God's answer agreeing to those terms. I immediately felt a peace and tranquility I couldn't explain.

In truth nothing had changed, but my perception of my dire situation was that I was no longer in mortal danger. I felt so confident that I didn't tell either of my two adult sons about the terminal diagnosis I had received. I didn't want to alarm them and have them believe in my imminent demise and give it power. They assumed I was fine, and I figured I had six months to find a way to break it to them if it turned out I wasn't. My oncology appointments soon became monthly events. My oncologist was kind and didn't scold me for basically doing nothing between the onset of my disease two years earlier and the awful new Stage IV diagnosis. She gave me a new prescription for Letrozole, the anti-estrogen drug. I didn't have much faith in it but lacking an alternative, I took it daily in the beginning. I knew if I was to survive, I had to believe there was a way out of this nightmare, even though the outcome looked very bad.

I took an initial assessment of myself and decided that I felt stronger in more areas than weak. Yes, I had cancer in my left hip and thigh, but not in the other side. My arms were cancer-free. I had cancer in one of my vertebrae, but not in any others. A small spot in my skull had not worked through to my brain. I considered these to be small victories. I either had a mass in my liver called a hemangioma, or it was cancer. They weren't sure which. A hemangioma was unlikely because it is a tangle of blood vessels that you're usually born with, and I knew that wasn't the case. I began to look for what I had been doing that caused me to get cancer twice within two years. Until I had it figured out, I decided to play by the cancer treatment rules. I became a good patient and followed some of the doctor's recommendations. I accepted a few low dose radiation treatments on one active spot in my cancer-ridden femur after my hip surgery. It was considered "palliative" therapy, and I only took 10 of the 15 recommended doses. I knew what palliative meant; that it was little more than a placebo. I took the outpatient rehabilitation services too, so I could learn to walk and bend down and put on my socks.

Because I had received a titanium hip replacement, my legs did not match in length anymore. My left leg was now about one-half inch longer than before, so I would have a permanent limp. It just made walking normally much harder, and more painful. I learned from my physical therapist that this is a common problem, but one I didn't expect. I used a cane, so I wouldn't look like I was about to tip over when I walked. Getting in and out of my small car was torturous, and I had to lift my left leg to get it inside and outside the car. I learned that lesson the first week I was home. I was instructed not to drive right away, and I was fine with that.

I made my debut to the outside world when my older sister who was in her 70's, but got around like a 30 something, drove the 60 miles between us to take me to lunch. I had to use a walker as I approached the restaurant because my left leg refused to support me when I walked. The place had double doors, which meant two people had to hold it open for me to enter. If either of them had let go, it would have knocked me down. It's unsettling to realize how fragile our bodies can become. It was a treat, and I was glad to see her, but because of the pain, I would have preferred to stay home. My surgically repaired left leg did not want to walk or work out. It wanted to sit on the couch and watch TV all day. It didn't care about sweeping the floor or standing to wash dishes or getting a shower. It was wounded and didn't want to obey orders from me or anyone else. When the laundry piled up and the floor grew dust bunnies, I tried to get busy, in a very slow, cautious way. Carrying laundry baskets across the floor was off limits but pushing them with a broom wasn't. Fortunately, I had the laundry room set up on the main floor. Sweeping wasn't so bad because I could use the broom as a cane as I moved across the floor. I cried a lot.

I had my first outpatient physical therapy appointment the second week after my hospital discharge. My physical therapists were very good at their jobs, if you count causing pain and suffering as a measurement. In the hospital, all I could accomplish was a few yards down the hallway with a walker. These pros expected much more from me. I felt like I was training for the Olympics. They had me bending my leg in ways it didn't want to bend: out to the side, outstretched front and back, climbing a staircase consisting of two then four stairs. Bending down was the worst part of any movement, and I was taught to throw out my left leg behind me whenever I had to reach down, in a sort of haphazard ballet move. It felt good, and I pretended that I was accomplishing my childhood dream of becoming a ballerina. I also was expected to sit on a stationary bike and pedal my legs for what seemed like hours but was really only 5 minutes. I was so proud when I finally progressed to 10 minutes, which I was able to do during the next two months.

I belong to the local YMCA, and it has a pool. I spent hours in it, gliding through the water, without limping, the water offering resistance that felt like an easy almost pain-free workout. The therapists recommended I use a pool at least once a week, and after a month, I was able to go back to work. The pain from the cancer had started to diminish, but the pain from the hip surgery had not.

At the hospital, the radiologist had decided there was no reason to radiate the cancer in my spine. It had invaded my T10 vertebra in my mid back and was about the size of the fingernail on my little finger. And it hurt. Both the oncologist and radiologist offered no treatment for my spine. That was frightening to me. I knew that if it continued to grow, I would eventually need surgery or become paralyzed, or both. It was 'wait and see time; let's see how bad this can get' time. Since my cancer was estrogen sensitive, this time I filled the prescription for the anti-estrogen hormone drug, Letrozole. The Letrozole would suppress estrogen production in the hope that it would slow down the cancer growth but was not expected to stop it.

The oncologist had told me that Letrozole "works" for about a year. "And then what?" I asked her. "Then we'll try something else" she said. I later learned that Letrozole helps delay further metastasis for only about 8 to 12 months. One newer drug, Ibrance, can help delay the spreading cancer about another 8 months on average. So, within two years, as a breast cancer patient, I could expect to have these medications stop working. Nowhere did it say I could expect the cancer to go away with either of them. I wasn't told if there was anything else, and I didn't have to ask. I knew there wasn't. Metastatic breast cancer patients have a median life span of thirty-six months. That means by year three, fifty percent of us have already died.

Currently, the five year survival rate is only 15% - 20%. My research also led me to the knowledge that even if someone dies from the cancer a few days after their five year mark, they consider them as five year survivors. That helps their statistics but most of these survivors are still not cancer free. Many have had it return, requiring other surgeries, more radiation treatments, chemo, and experimental treatments. Few if any, apparently, can say the cancer is gone for good. The therapies or meds stop working after a while, and the cancer keeps rearing its ugly head. Sometimes cancer patients end up with multiple types of cancer, as happened to my father, who first got prostate cancer, then colon cancer. I myself have had skin cancer, basal cell and squamous cell, as well as the breast cancer and all occurring within the same time frame.

Hope, I have learned, is the foundation of survival. I have observed that people, including myself, do not pay attention to alternative voices, they don't do further research, or make the changes necessary to survive, if they don't believe they can be helped. If you put all your trust in the medical professionals, you may likely end up disappointed like I was. I know the fear and panic of being told you might not survive very much longer. Every day people give up hope because they have reached the limits of current medical treatment for the disease they are fighting. Or their hope has been misplaced because it was based on old and useless treatments that don't work for them, and in fact make their condition much, much worse. It was hope that guided my research and kept me going through those first few weeks, with the idea of dying gradually fading from my thoughts. When I was looking online and reading books and magazines, I was able to keep those morbid thoughts away. I never lost hope, and I believe that's why I persisted and kept praying and looking for answers until I found them.

I started reading everything online and in magazines I could find about natural remedies. Most articles I read focused on one particular supplement or food to eat or avoid. I collected many different pieces of information that I hoped would help in my recovery. I decided to try the ones that seemed legitimate. Most were inexpensive and almost none of them required a prescription. They also didn't have a long list of potentially deadly side effects.

The doctors offer a treatment plan, and without an alternative, most meekly agree with it. According to the doctor who treated me, I was going to die from Stage IV Breast Cancer by the end of 2015.

I'm glad he told me that. If he had offered me false hope, I might not have relied on other resources. I can say that most of what I believe helped me survive was not the advice I received from my doctors. Those in the medical field are caught up in doing what's been done for decades, even though the results are terrible for most cancer patients.

If your life is on the line and you are facing a serious bout of cancer, then you have to become your own advocate. Ask your doctor for advice, but ask about how effective those treatments are statistically. Ask about potential side effects. Ask about alternatives with fewer side effects. Then do some serious research on more natural alternatives. The more information you have, the better your chances of survival become.

Chapter 2:
Why is Cancer so Puzzling?

I thought it might help me fight cancer if I understood it better so part of my research involved getting to know more about it. I already knew that cancer is essentially an overgrowth of your own body cells. I wanted to find out why they become rogue cells that spiral out of control. In "Health Basics: The True History of Cancer in the USA", author S.D. Wells defines cancer as "the uncontrolled division, multiplication and spread of mutated and warped calls that attack healthy cells and organs." But why does our body turn on us? What causes it? "Most cancer stems from the consumption of chemicals that cause an acidic body to be deprived of oxygen and nutrients" according to the article. It blames the "toxic food and medicine environment" for the current statistic of one in three Americans who get cancer. He cites radiation and chemotherapy drugs, mercury in vaccines, aluminum in flu shots as examples of toxic medicines. He also claims sodium fluoride added to our water supply is a toxic chemical. I found another article titled "Cancer Develops from Fungal Infections like Candida" on NaturalNews.com. The author, Derek Henry, states that a systemic fungal infection can be brought on by "antibiotics, birth control pills, excessive sugar and grain consumption, chemicals that mimic estrogen in the body, alcohol, smoking, and heavy metals." The largest contributor to candida in our bodies is sugar. Other causes include pesticides used on our food, polluted drinking water, dental fillings, hormone therapies and prescription drugs.

According to the article, a Nobel Prize was awarded to Otto Warburg in 1931 for informing the world that oxygen is the enemy of cancer. Once in the blood stream, candida takes over certain areas of the body and reduces oxygen levels. Candida grows unchecked in this unhealthy internal environment. So do cancer cells. The result is an unhealthy intestinal ecology where bacteria, yeast, fungi, and mold grow and transform cells from a healthy to an unhealthy state. Beneficial bacteria in your gut do not work well when overrun by candida. Cancer can be caused by or in conjunction with a fungal infection, according to the author. It often then takes years for cancers to develop.

If you have a "sweet tooth" and crave sugar or alcohol, you probably have an overgrowth of candida in your system. John Hopkins Hospital found that the drug "itraconazole, which is commonly used to treat toenail fungus, can also block angiogenesis, or the growth of new blood vessels commonly seen in cancers, which allow metastases to occur", according to the article. Eliminating sweets and harmful chemicals and taking an antifungal medication can help eliminate candida from your body and reduce the growth of cancer cells. Probiotics help balance your intestinal bacteria as well. There are over the counter yeast fighting supplements at your health food store as well.

So far in this chapter, I have referenced articles that focus on how people can become exposed to cancer-causing agents. While there appear to be many causes, cancer risks and prevention are not very popular topics it seems. Why is it you rarely see TV ads that warn you about cancer causing chemicals sprayed on our crops? It seems the only ones running are ads to let you know about class-action lawsuits against the manufacturers of specific cancer causing chemicals, but they are only from attorneys aimed at people already diagnosed.

I found an online article I think explains this phenomenon. It points out that most cancer research doesn't focus on the prevention and causes of cancer. The focus instead is on finding a cure once you already have it. I read "Cancer Researchers Don't Want a Cure, They Would Lose Billions" on Newstarget.com. What I learned is that cancer researchers like to stress genetic testing as a way to identify your likelihood of getting a certain type of cancer. But only a small percentage of cancer cases can be attributed to genetic mutations from our parents. Yet research is focused heavily on genetic causes essentially to avoid focusing on the toxins that cause the majority of cancer cases. All the money spent, and research done over the last fifty years has had very little impact on cancer. In fact, it is more prevalent now than it was decades ago. Earlier detection can account for a small increase in five-year survival rates. With such little progress, it would seem likely that they don't really want to find a cancer cure. I had to read the article again before a light bulb went off in my head. Then it was more like a nuclear bomb exploding in my mind. Suddenly, all the hope, caring and compassion that's displayed on TV, along with the pleading for donations to help find a cure didn't ring true to me.

Have we been conned all along? Why would that be? Could it be possible that people in the medical field would actually have no interest in trying to find a cure or educate us on potential causes? Once I considered the possibility, I had to see where that train of thought led me. Sadly, I began to believe it could be true. The Newstarget.com article explained that much of the very expensive ongoing cancer research is funded by donations from large corporations. Some of those large corporations produce and sell toxic products. In exchange for their dollars, the cancer researchers protect them from scrutiny by diverting our attention to an elusive cure they're just about to find or a genetic cause that doesn't apply to most of us.

But why would they thwart efforts to save our lives? The answer is evident when you follow the money. In addition to donations from these corporations, the medical community depends on long term consumers. Oncologists, surgeons, nurses, radiologists, physical therapists, technicians and hospitals rely on a steady stream of cancer patients. If cancer was cured or prevented on a large scale, they would lose their ever-increasing profits. That would affect their bottom line, their real priority. I really don't want to think that so many lives, including mine, could be so cheaply regarded.

Yet, the treatments they offer aren't designed to cure us, but to prolong our lives as sick patients requiring a never ending series of treatments. The side effects are debilitating so pain management becomes an important part of our treatment plan, enabling the drug companies to enjoy tremendous profits too.

Cancer treatment is a multibillion-dollar industry and the survival rate for Stage IV cancer patients is very dismal. Nobody expects modern cancer treatments to be very successful in providing a cancer cure, especially when it's at the Stage IV metastatic - worst possible diagnosis you can get - level. Unless it's been caught very early, cancer is hard to cure with today's medical products. Even then, there's no guarantee. A cancer is cured when all traces of it are removed from the patient's body. Five years of remission is the benchmark for success. It's easier to live for five years if it doesn't reach the Stage IV phase where it has spread to other parts of the body, like the lungs, bones, and liver. Of course, even after the chemo, radiation, and drugs, if you don't make changes that caused it in the first place, it is very likely to come back. But who tells you that?

I can't be sure, but I suspect more than half of

all cancer patients don't search for alternative cancer cures. Or if they do, for the most part they don't believe they should follow an alternative path because their doctors will discourage them from trying something they can't get from a hospital, pharmacy, or doctor's office. I felt this was the case when I asked Dr. B. for information about possible causes. He claimed not to know, and even denied the risk of aluminum in antiperspirants even though I found research supporting the idea. He didn't advise me to stop using it or to do anything differently.

I began to understand how cancer patients and their caregivers become almost totally dependent on their medical team when facing this monster of a disease. Their doctors warn them against trying alternative non-medical options, and label people who support these options as frauds, but won't warn them against sugar. Patients are led to believe their physicians must know what's best for them. Just because they have a treatment plan for cancer patients that in most cases is the same one-size-fits-all plan, doesn't mean it's actually effective. You need to be aware that no one cares more about your recovery than you do. I didn't trust my recovery to physicians, especially after I was told I was going to die in the not-too-distant future. If I wanted to survive, I had to be a pioneer, a researcher, even a guinea pig. Eventually, I considered myself lucky I was told they couldn't cure me. It gave me the freedom to explore alternatives they wouldn't approve of, with none of the pressure to try any more of theirs.

Chapter 3:
Going "Au Naturel"

Shortly after my terminal cancer diagnosis, I started with something I did have faith in; natural, non-prescription options. I have had an interest in vitamins and alternative natural therapies for many years, starting after a prescribed blood pressure medication gave me a bad case of tinnitus. Tinnitus is hard to deal with, especially when it's new and it causes a very loud ringing in your ears. It means you never get to be in a silent room again. To my dismay, I learned that there was no cure for me, even after stopping the medication. The only remedy I found after consulting with two ENT (Ears-Nose-Throat) doctors was to avoid loud sounds, use white noise from a radio to fall asleep to, and avoid salt. Salt raises blood pressure and apparently affects the blood flow in your ears which makes the noise louder. I found CoQ10 helped lower my blood pressure and it was cheaper than the BP meds and didn't cause side effects. So, it was natural for me to start my belated research on cancer with vitamins and supplements in mind.

I tried to recall what I had heard about alternative treatments for cancer. I remembered reading several years ago about Vitamin B17 or Laetrile, as it is also called. It was banned in the U.S. decades ago, because people were using it instead of chemotherapy for cancer. It was very controversial at the time with the medical community saying it was fake and not effective and a threat to the people who were taking it since they were not taking chemotherapy as they should be. The people who wanted to take Laetrile were arguing that the FDA banned it because it was effective as a cancer cure and a threat to the standard cancer protocol.

Vitamin B17 occurs naturally in the seeds of apricots and peaches. But it has to be carefully processed. According to "Laetrile Cancer Research Cover-up" on mercola.com, laetrile is the patented drug made from the natural compound in the seeds of apricots and peaches. Laetrile contains glucose, benzaldehyde, and cyanide. Cyanide is believed to be the anti-cancer compound, because it's toxic to all cells, but more toxic to cancer cells than normal ones. It's very unlikely that a person would get cyanide poisoning from laetrile because of very low levels involved, according to the article. Even if it is effective, I would have to travel to Mexico to get it, because it's still banned here in the U.S. There is an alternative way to get Vitamin B17 that I found in my online search. Apparently, it occurs naturally in millet, an ancient, gluten-free grain. You can buy millet bread in health food stores. I have never tried it, but it may be a better alternative to wheat bread.

It took me plenty of research and dogged persistence to put all the cancer killing puzzle pieces together. I found a British Medical Journal's online article "Higher Vitamin D Levels may be Linked to Lower Risk of Cancer" about a Japanese study on Vitamin D levels. Their conclusion was that taking high levels of about 2000 IUs of Vitamin D daily can decrease your relative risk of overall cancer by about 20%. I was elated to find that study, but also puzzled. For me, 20% is a small but significant statistic. Some people might look at those results and conclude that Vitamin D really won't make much difference, so why bother? I hung onto that 20% statistic as if it were a lifeline. I had to ask myself though, what about the other 80% of people in the study where higher levels of Vitamin D made no difference? Why didn't it? I couldn't find a conclusive answer from that summary.

The Japanese study followed thousands of men and women from the year 2000 to 2009. Some of the participants had developed cancers of the colon, liver, breast and prostate during that time. The researchers concluded that low levels of the vitamin were found to be associated with the spread of cancer. The study supported the hypothesis that high Vitamin D levels may have beneficial effects in preventing cancer, but that the protection has a ceiling effect, in that there are no additional benefits beyond a certain level of the vitamin.

Because I had more questions about Vitamin D and its role in cancer, I kept looking for other articles. None of the studies I looked at concluded that low vitamin D levels actually caused cancer. But at least one other study stated that low levels may help cancer to spread, particularly to the bones. A 2011 WebMD online article with the title "Low Vitamin D levels linked to Advanced Cancers" concluded that the vitamin helps regulate genes that keep cancer cells from spreading. Vitamin D also helps regulate calcium which is responsible for healthy bones.

So far, I had found two sources that concluded that low Vitamin D levels were associated with cancer progression. Since cancer can grow and spread when Vitamin D levels are low, I wondered what my levels were. I suspected they were low, so I asked my oncologist for a blood test during the next monthly visit. I didn't know if there was a problem with my Vitamin D levels since I was already taking one 400 I.U. capsule of Vitamin D daily. My Vitamin D levels were low, and breast cancer cells had been spreading to my bones. My doctor recommended I take 2,000 I.U.s a day, which was the only non-medical advice I have received from her.

The next question I researched was whether high Vitamin D blood levels can actually reverse cancer progression. The online article "Is Vitamin D the New Silver Bullet for Cancer?" says that it has been shown to do so. I was elated to read that test results on mice injected with Vitamin D showed cancer tumors shrinking more than fifty percent in a few weeks. I was very thankful to find evidence that my cancer maybe, possibly, would reverse itself if there were higher levels of Vitamin D in my system. But none of the studies, including that one, showed that cancer in the mice or in humans was eliminated by adding Vitamin D alone. But it was an important piece of the puzzle I had to solve.

After doing lots more research with somewhat similar statistics on individual compounds (vitamins, minerals, supplements, foods, etc.) I came to the conclusion that there must be a synergistic effect. That is, the participants who benefitted from the Vitamin D study must have been adding other things to their diet and at the same time eliminating exposure to harmful substances that the majority wasn't. I can't say for sure that's how it worked for them, but I used that idea as a hypothesis and found it to work for my own cancer recovery. It was a Eureka moment for me every time the medical tests I underwent showed that my own cancer spots and suspected cancer spots were shrinking and then just disappearing. I knew I had my answer.

Chapter 4:
I Believe I Can Survive

I began to believe I had a chance to survive, if only for a little while longer. I decided to have faith that natural remedies weren't all bogus. I made the changes in my lifestyle and my diet that I read could possibly save my life. I had no guarantee of success by following these recommendations because there was no one I could ask "Hey, how'd that work out for you?" I am here to tell you, it worked. What I learned and put into practice allowed me to live and get healthy again. It's wonderful to wake up every morning without counting down how many days I have left.

As a Geriatric Social Worker, I had worked many years helping senior citizens who were nearing the end of their lives. Many of them developed cancer and were given the usual surgery, radiation, and chemo routine. I visited them in nursing homes, consulted with their medical teams about surgical procedures and medications they needed, and helped them make burial arrangements. I attended their funerals and hugged their family members when they died. I did the same with my friends and family members I lost to cancer. Even with the best of care given to them, their cancers never left them for long, and they all died. I knew that same fate awaited me unless I did something different than they had.

One thing they all had in common was that they all took chemotherapy. My friends, family members, and some clients had all said "Yes" when it was offered to them. So that's where I started, by saying "No". I am not a paid researcher, but I acted like one. What I stumbled over in my search for a cure was a series of clues that I experimented with as if my life depended on it, because it did.

I stopped taking the Letrozole after the pain from the cancer started to retreat. I still had fragile femur bones where the cancer was because my bones were leaching calcium into my bloodstream. To combat that, my oncologist suggested that I take an Xgeva shot monthly. It helps draw calcium from your bloodstream back into your bones but carries some risks. For instance, I could have my jaw bone disintegrate from a tooth extraction up to ten years from the Xgeva shots. I stopped the Xgeva shots for elevated calcium in my bloodstream because of new tests ordered and interpreted by an ENT doctor that indicated my slightly elevated calcium wasn't a response to cancer, but a reaction to a parathyroid gland that's overactive. So, I had hyperparathyroidism too.

Hyperparathyroidism can cause high blood pressure, high calcium levels, atrial fibrillation, and high cholesterol. I had all of those. The only cure, I was told, was surgical removal of my one rogue parathyroid gland. I was anxious to have this threat to my health removed, so I agreed. It was a disaster. The surgeon removed half my thyroid gland during the surgery in a failed attempt to find the enlarged parathyroid. So, I was not any better off, and in fact I was worse off because now I also had to deal with low thyroid levels as well. Symptoms include achiness, hair loss, and extreme tiredness, but my doctor refused to give me any medicine because my blood levels didn't warrant thyroid replacement drugs. That's probably a good thing, because once again I turned to natural alternatives that provided symptom relief.

I found that thyroid supplements and kelp tablets helped. I also took zinc and iodine drops my son found for me online which has helped the most. It's from Go Nutrients and called "Iodine Edge" drops. I added Vitamin K2 which helps regulate calcium in the blood and has helped reduce my parathyroid hormone levels by hundreds of points to near normal. As a result, my parathyroid hormone levels dropped from over 600 to 198, still slightly high, but I no longer have heart palpitations. My risk of stroke or heart attack has greatly diminished. Taking Vitamins K2 has helped relieve all of those issues by regulating my parathyroid hormone. I also added Vitamin K1 which is different from Vitamin K2. K1 helps with blood clotting and is found in leafy green vegetables. Vitamin K2 helps direct calcium into bones and out of soft tissues like kidneys and arteries. Of course, this is something I found out from my own research without anyone in the medical field sharing this very important non-medical information with me.

Why does it seem they only share information about therapies they can make a profit from? I was able to stop the exorbitantly priced Xgeva shots which costs over $2,000 each and comes with serious health risks. I had more than twelve of them before I found an effective alternative in Vitamins K1 and K2. Fortunately, the health risks from my hyperparathyroidism were eliminated and because I was able to use natural remedies to do so, it gave me even more incentive to keep looking for a natural cancer healing as well.

My attitude about becoming a cancer patient was formed years before I got diagnosed with the disease. Several years back while working on the side as a life insurance agent, I met a woman in her early 40's with young children who had already had surgery to remove her lower left leg due to cancer. At that point, I could not sell her a policy and her family had no funds set aside to pay for her cremation when she died a few months later. That lady reminded me of a promise I made to myself many years ago.

When I was 19, I saw the movie "Love Story". It was released in 1970, and starred Ryan O'Neal and Ali McGraw. It had a lifelong impact on my attitude toward cancer treatment. In the movie, Ali's character "Jenny" is diagnosed with a terminal disease (the book says it's leukemia) and has a choice to either take chemo or something similar, and live about nine more months in agony or die quicker without it. Jenny decides to skip the chemo and die with all her hair and body parts. I decided that was a brave choice I would make under the same conditions. Her famous line to her movie husband "Love means never having to say you're sorry" comes after he apologizes for getting angry, and it puzzled me for years. What did she mean by that statement? I don't know what the intent was in the movie, but for me it means that I don't want to have to say "I'm sorry" to myself for using a futile and painful poisonous treatment that would kill me anyway or lose a limb to try to save the rest of my body for a while longer. Surgery can help but losing limbs to cancer surgery can be traumatic.

I also don't want to be sorry for withholding information about my recovery that could help others. I believe we should share our God given gifts to others with love. It pains me greatly to know others are suffering and dying or have died from cancer when they might otherwise have lived.

Chapter 5:
Why I Don't Believe
in Chemotherapy

Many people choose chemotherapy and I often wonder why. Since I told them upfront I wouldn't take it, I never got the sales pitch from the doctors. What is it they say to make people want to burn their insides out? I was already on a path leading to more intense pain, immobility, hospice and certain death, all within six months. I didn't need the sickness, pain and chronic side effects from chemo on top of all that.

When you have a cancer diagnosis, and the outlook looks grim, you have choices to make. Should you agree to radiation? Chemotherapy? Surgery? When your life is on the line, does it make sense to blindly follow the path a doctor sets for you? Can you justify following the medical protocol of surgery, radiation and chemo without knowing if they're even effective? I had the opportunity to talk with nurses and technicians at the hospital during the several tests I underwent the first year after my terminal diagnosis. It's amazing what you can find out just by being friendly with them. On one occasion I was told that some of the wheelchair patients who come routinely for their chemo infusions are not really going to benefit from them, it just makes them feel like the hospital staff and doctors are doing something for them. It kind of gives them a little hope, but it's really not doing anything to help them, it just makes them sicker.

The decisions you make initially may determine later whether you live or die. When they tell you chemo will help you live longer, ask them for some statistics on that. If they admit that there is nothing further that medical science can do for you, will you just give up? Will you just sit around and wait to die? The answer to these questions for me was a most definite "No!" The reason I decided to go without chemo was also based on my observation of other cancer victims who have died from the disease after receiving standard medical care. After witnessing the relentless progression of cancer on friends and family members who went through chemotherapy and ultimately died, I felt chemo would just make all the horrors of this disease worse for me as it sadly did for them.

For some people, the long-term consequences of this treatment can be almost as bad as the cancer. Because cancer cells tend to multiply fast, chemo drugs target fast growing cells, even non-cancerous ones. They can damage cells in the heart, kidneys, lungs, and nervous system, causing long term damage to those organs and others including the bladder. Nerve damage like tingling and pain may be long lasting and difficult to live with. Chemo was what my doctors recommended for me, but I was unwilling to deal with the side effects. Chemo and radiation do nothing to treat the root cause of cancer, so they are not cures, only treatments. Their effectiveness is something even the medical staff find questionable.

Doing something different saved my life. I want people I may never meet who are struggling with their own personal or family cancer tragedy to have access to the same information that has kept me alive. In 2016, during the first year of my remission, I spoke with an old neighbor, someone dealing with a different kind of cancer that happened to be very aggressive. At the time, she looked healthy and was in her early 60's like me. I briefly told her and her husband about what I was doing to heal my cancer and my decision to avoid chemotherapy and the success I was having. The treatment plan her doctor gave her unfortunately included chemotherapy, but they felt optimistic about her future. I lost contact with them until recently, when I heard of her death from the cancer through an acquaintance. She died in intensive care, just after taking what would be her last infusion of chemo drugs she felt she needed. Her copays for chemo I learned later added up to several thousand dollars a month. It was heartbreaking for me to learn of this tragedy. Sadly, it wasn't an unexpected outcome to me.

Chemo doesn't just destroy cancer cells. I learned a lot by watching a YouTube video called "Chemo and Radiation Treatment Does NOT Work 97% of The Time". In the video Dr. Leonard Coldwell gives this analogy: "If you have a garden with flowers and bushes and trees and grass, and some weeds, you come with Agent Orange and kill it all off, and now it's all dead, and you hope only the good stuff is coming back" Coldwell says. "They bombard the entire system and then they say the cancer is in remission. For three years, you have no cancer, you're cured. You're just dead in five years." Chemo is like weed killer, but it doesn't discriminate. It kills healthy cells too. Just as healthy cells come back, so do the cancer cells.

I also had five other good reasons to skip chemo: my father, uncle, sister, nephew, and cousin all died from cancer after going through grueling chemotherapy. If I had only known then what I know now, perhaps they would still be here. But hope and a cure came too late for the cancer victims in my family. People I loved suffered and died after putting all their faith and trust in the medical professionals who treated them. In the end, after all the radiation, chemo and surgery they endured, none of it worked. They each died a slow and painful death after a short time in remission. People like my sister Shirley who was diagnosed with Multiple Myeloma, a bone marrow cancer, during the same week we buried my father. She spent the following eight years of her life trying to overcome cancer with surgery, radiation, chemo and bone marrow transplants. She went to the best hospitals in Florida. It kept coming back. I spoke to her by phone a few days before she died. I asked if the latest bone-marrow transplant had put her in remission. She said it hadn't. Less than a week later, I got the call she was gone.

Let me tell you that metastatic breast cancer and other cancers can be very painful. My sister was in severe pain for years due to the cancer and chemo. She never complained and always kept her cheerful and loving attitude, but it showed on her face. She knew up until the end that she was going to die from it. My father died from colon cancer in 1995. His cancer treatment consisted of progressive radiation, chemotherapy, and surgery to remove parts of his colon. His medical care included a colostomy bag. He was bed-ridden and on morphine for months before succumbing to this awful disease.

My wonderful nephew Douglas died at the young age of 47 in 2015 from melanoma shortly after my hip surgery. My cousin Kenny died of lung cancer in 2016. I never had the chance to tell them about my recovery. All of them followed medical advice and standard treatment including surgery, radiation and chemo, and they all died painfully slow deaths. None of these expensive treatments worked for them. I wish I could go back in time and tell each of them to take precautions before they got cancer. My sister in Florida had the worst toxic looking water coming from her kitchen sink, but she used it for coffee and cooking anyway. It was so dirty that I could not drink it while visiting her on vacation. She also worked in a large warehouse full of chemicals.

My father had a sugar addiction and would eat a whole gallon of ice cream in one sitting. He was overweight for most of his life. My nephew was light skinned and blonde and worked and played in the sun without sunscreen for most of his life. Skin cancer grew on his back, where it wasn't found until it had metastasized. My cousin Kenny was a chain smoker and heavy alcohol user. Today we know there is a connection between smoking, alcohol, chemicals in our air and water, sun exposure, and bad diet. Most people believe it won't happen to them, until it does. There are steps you can take to help prevent cancer but lots of people don't quit smoking even after they have throat or lung cancer or need an oxygen tank. Although I had previously smoked cigarettes, I quit after thirteen years, at age thirty. Alcohol was not part of my life, other than an occasional glass of wine. I did not feel either of those substances were responsible for my breast cancer, because too many years had passed. I could not however, rule out a bad diet as a factor.

Chapter 6:
From Cancer Patient
to Cancer Survivor

There is a wealth of information out there that helped me survive. I wasn't getting enough information from the doctors and I was determined to find out the "why" of my cancer and how to overcome it if possible. I read about the Budwig diet for cancer in several articles and on their website, "BudwigCenter.com" about cottage cheese and flaxseed. I tried it and found it filling and a good substitute for empty calories. I studied the acidic vs. the alkaline diet. An article online titled "Can a Low-Acid Diet Help Prevent Cancer?" states that "alkaline foods such as fresh fruits, vegetables, nuts, legumes and root vegetables …nourish good bacteria in your gut…that help decrease inflammation throughout the body that might otherwise contribute to cancer". On the other hand, foods such as refined sugar and flour and animal fat create an acidic environment in your gut because they are difficult to digest. It's possible these foods can contribute to cancer. They can contribute to candida overgrowth in your intestinal tract. When I looked at the food I was eating, including processed meats like bacon and lunch meats, TV dinners, biscuits and breads, I could see how they may have contributed to my cancer. Armed with new information, I made significant changes to my diet, threw out my aluminum containing antiperspirant, and stopped the black cohosh. I bought different supplements, herbs and vitamins based on my research and started taking them religiously. I stopped eating ice cream, donuts, and cookies and started eating salads and lean chicken and fish.

I lost fifty-five pounds. I should mention I got a jump start on my diet in the hospital. The smell of hospital food made me nauseous, so for eight days, I had no solid food. The yeast in bread was a smell that made me sick, so bread was not in my diet for months and I seldom eat it now. Yeast and fungi are related and are associated with cancer risk. I found supplements that were possibly helpful in reducing cancer risk, and chemicals that were additives in processed food to avoid.

After the physical therapy ended, I continued to exercise regularly at the YMCA. I could not do strenuous exercise, but I could work out lightly on a treadmill and stationary bike. Regular exercise can help you lose weight and reduce body fat, which is important in your recovery. After eliminating pork from my diet, I noticed I had less joint stiffness. I took glucosamine for arthritis in my neck and spine and became much more limber and pain free. When it comes to surviving cancer, knowledge really is power.

I have been to the oncology department of our local hospital many times over the last six years for regular checkups. In May of 2017, at a scheduled three-month office visit with my oncologist, I reminded her of it being the second anniversary of my terminal cancer diagnosis. Out of curiosity, I asked her, "How am I doing compared to your other patients? I mean, how many of your patients besides me are in remission at their two year mark?" Her answer stunned me. "You're the only one", she said. "What?" I blurted out loud. That was all I could think to say. Then she started to explain about overall remission statistics being about fifteen percent but did not change her answer that I was the only one of her patients to be in remission at the two year mark. I felt scared and sad when she told me that, especially when she said the younger women don't do as well as us older ones. She has a very busy practice and treats cancer patients of all ages. Some women with young children were dying or already dead. It was a horrific revelation to me, and one that still haunts me. As a mother, there is nothing more important in my life than raising my children to be successful and happy adults. I imagine most mothers feel the same.

The oncology office has a chemo station where several patients can sit while receiving a slow drip of drugs into their veins, and I have observed them sitting there tethered to the plastic lines that end in a port in their skin. I've seen many women coming in, appearing weak, being pushed in wheelchairs, and with scarves covering their bald heads. I shudder to think that could have been me. I have always been able to walk through the hospital to the oncology department, at first with a walker, then a cane and now, without assistance.

At year two and a half, CT scans of my kidney and liver showed only remnants of the prior suspected cancer, calling them non-cancerous "cysts." There was no mention of the suspected hemangioma which, had it been a hemangioma, would not have disappeared. I have learned to walk with little to no hint of a limp. I cannot run, but at least I am pain free. These changes from cancerous to normal occurred without any medical treatment at all, except for the initial three months of

Letrozole and a few initial "palliative" radiation treatments on my thigh. The doctor who delivered my cancer diagnosis in my hospital room in 2015 believed in my imminent death. For a while, it seemed likely. But every day the symptoms lessened. The pain eventually went away. The tests showed I was winning the battle. The cancer was receding. It is now gone. So far, I have won the fight.

I never shared with my doctor any of the diet and supplemental regimen I have imposed on myself. I just felt it would be pointless. Periodically, she orders tests, like CT scans, bone scans, X-rays, brain scans and others to chart the progression of my disease. I have refused the bone scans and brain scans in the last two years because they carry their own risks. Following those tests, I developed a noticeable short term memory loss which has not gone away completely. When the tests showed the cancer was shrinking, she felt that the Letrozole, the anti-estrogen pill, was the reason. I never disagreed with her about it, because it may have helped for the first three months that I took it. Letrozole, she explained, only inhibits the amount of estrogen in the body, so is only effective for estrogen sensitive cancers like I had. It works to stop or slow down cancer but only for a very limited time before the cancer rebounds. It also only works if and while you are taking it. I stopped it four years ago.

Women with early stage breast cancer treated with Letrozole following surgery fared far better than late Stage IV users like me. One study from 2007 on the National Institute of Health website "Letrozole in advanced breast cancer" showed that the median time to progression of tumor growth for Letrozole users was nine months. The median survival for the Letrozole group was thirty-five months. Letrozole also causes osteoporosis, bone fractures, pain, and a host of other side effects, and some of the women in the trial dropped out of the study because of these side effects. I've already survived longer than I would have if I had continued with the Letrozole.

After being diagnosed and treated for cancer, I became disappointed in the cancer treatment industry. Initially the surgeries I had reduced the cancer in my body but did not keep it from spreading. I know the small amount of radiation they offered, and I eventually accepted, may lead to future cancers. I believe the chemotherapy would not have stopped cancer because it doesn't work for most people long term, and it didn't work for people I love who died in spite of or because of it. I think doctors could and should have done more to educate me and others on how to keep it from spreading further. I have read that chemo makes them on average over a million dollars per patient if they live at least a year. It's easy to be critical and conclude that these cancer treatments do more for doctors than they do for us patients.

The cancer industry appears to want to perpetuate cancer care, because treatment is very lucrative for them, and a cure might cause the industry to collapse. That's not just my opinion either. In an article online from 2014 in Health Impact News, author John P. Thomas writes "They want us to stop asking the question, 'Why has the 40-year war on cancer failed to produce any results?' They want us to stop asking why there are only three approved treatments for cancer (surgery, radiation therapy, and chemo-therapy) and why no new cancer therapies have been approved by the US FDA in the last one hundred years. They want us to have hope for a brighter day in cancer treatment while our friends and family die by the thousands every day." His article is titled: "Cancer Makes Too Much Money to Cure" and lists the medical costs of cancer treatment at $125 billion as of 2014. Since 2014, there has been a flurry of cancer drugs approved by the FDA, but most do little or nothing to improve cancer survival rates, according to a USA Today report of 2/9/2017. The report titled "Dozens of New Cancer Drugs do little to Improve Survival" says that in addition, these drugs come with risks and side effects and cost an average of $171,000 per year.

Another important point is the financial toll that cancer can have on your life. If you receive a cancer diagnosis and can't work for an extended period of time, you will likely have financial difficulties. I assumed I could get help from cancer charities that are always raising money for cancer victims. I was surprised to learn that it isn't their primary goal. They mostly raise money for research. However, of the billion dollars raised by the American Cancer Society each year, more than sixty percent goes to pay their staff. Another fifteen percent goes to pay for mailers and advertising to raise more money. That leaves twenty-five percent for cancer research.

Contributions made to the American Cancer Society do not go to help cancer victims directly, except for rides to treatment and lodging near treatment centers. That's not much to give to cancer victims, most of whom have their own transportation to their local medical appointments. When I was diagnosed with Stage IV Breast Cancer and unable to work for a month, I got behind on utility bills. When I got a disconnect notice on my electric bill, I called the American Cancer Society for help. To my surprise, they said they don't help individuals with those kinds of problems. They gave me the number for another nonprofit agency who said I had to fill out an application and supply medical records. They agreed to pay one bill. That was their limit. They paid the past due amount on my electric bill which stopped the disconnection. However, they didn't pay the current amount due, so a month later, I was behind again. I called other nonprofits but since I got help from one agency, they would not even give me an application. I had no choice but to go back to work when I could still barely walk. I was lucky I still had a job. Later I found out that a Stage IV cancer diagnosis is pretty much an automatic qualifier for Social Security Disability benefits, but it takes six months to process.

Chapter 7:
What is the Cost of a
Pound of Sugar?

To me, the price of sugar is much too high to pay, no matter how cheap it is. It's a killer if you have cancer. In the 2012 book, "Cancer as a Metabolic Disease" by Dr. Thomas Seyfried, the author sums it up this way: "No real progress has been made in the management of advanced or metastatic cancer for more than 40 years." Essentially, he is saying your chance of surviving metastatic cancer is the same as it was decades ago. Dr. Seyfried explains that "Cancer cells depend largely on glucose and glutamine metabolism for survival." That means when sugar is unavailable to nourish them, cancer cells will die. This is very important information for anyone who has cancer to memorize and put into practice. Sugar feeds cancer. If you starve cancer, it will die. I have reason to believe this is true. Changing my diet to eliminate added sugar, including corn syrup, has, I believe, significantly helped to keep cancer at bay.

Is it any coincidence that overall cancer rates are up when sugar is inserted into almost all of our processed food? The food industry knows sugar is highly addictive. Despite the risk of obesity, diabetes, yeast infections and cancer, the majority of people in this country won't give it up. Is it a coincidence with our modern diet that just about one in three people will get cancer in their lifetime? If I had looked into the diet and cancer connection earlier, I might never have had my breast cancer develop from Stage II to Stage IV in two years. Your doctor probably won't tell you that cakes, donuts, pasta and alcohol are feeding your cancer cells. Nothing about diet was even mentioned to me by any of the various doctors or specialists I consulted during the first years after my cancer diagnosis, until I asked about it.

When I decided I was not going to let cancer kill me, I asked as many questions as I could think of when I went back to the hospital for different kinds of tests. One body scan early after my Stage IV diagnosis searched and found cancer cells in my body after I drank a sugary liquid with dye in it. When I asked why they used sugar to find cancer cells in the body, the technician told me that cancer cells light up in the presence of sugar. Sugar makes cancer cells grow and cancer cells absorb sugar as fast as possible. Cancer cells react "like pouring gasoline onto a fire", he said. He also said, "They know that", meaning the cancer doctors. And they had given it to me for this test, and it showed where I had cancer residing in my body, like my left hip area, thigh and vertebra. Why didn't any doctor tell me? I couldn't get that question out of my head. They obviously knew. If I hadn't asked that technician, I may not have found out in time.

So, I had learned about a giant piece of the cancer puzzle. Cancer cells feed directly on our food. When you eat sugary foods, you are growing more cancer cells. Sugar is addictive. I see a pattern here. I had to ask myself, why was he the first person to tell me this? Cancer cells grow exponentially with sugar for fuel. I believed him because this was a medical technician telling me so. And what if I hadn't asked? I was horrified to know I might have continued to feed cancer, knowing where it would have led me. After all, I had kept eating sugar for almost two years after my initial diagnosis, and it metastasized to my hip and other areas. I wouldn't have lived another two years. I made an immediate change in my diet. I decided to stop eating sugar, even though none of the hospital staff, not the doctors, radiologists, nurses or even the technician advised me to do so. None of the free cancer magazines at the hospital that tell you to be a good, compliant patient and get plenty of rest after your chemo drip tell us cancer patients to reduce or eliminate sugar. Unbelievable! They all know that sugar feeds cancer cells, but no one on my medical team would recommend that I stop it. I still don't have an answer as to why this information isn't posted on highway billboards.

I can be kind and assume that maybe they think cancer patients wouldn't listen anyway. It pains me to see a dear friend of mine who is also a cancer patient eating sugary desserts after telling me about her chemo pills and infusion schedule. Although I have mentioned that sugar is detrimental to her recovery, she has not changed her diet and her cancer has spread throughout her body. She is unable to walk because it is in both of her femurs.

Increasing the odds of survival from cancer depends on making lifestyle changes that may be hard to do. You may be addicted to sugar, like lots of people are. It's not hopeless though. People don't have to be slaves to sugar addiction. It's vital to overall health to eliminate sugar and reduce carbs and alcohol which converts to sugar in your system. You'll feel healthier and it's good to feel free of an addiction as powerful as sugar. The good news is you don't have to use willpower alone to conquer a sugar addiction. There is a medication you can get from your doctor to curb your sugar cravings. It's called Terbinafine. There are others but that's the one I was prescribed. It's an anti-fungal tablet and it kills candida. Sugar feeds candida overgrowth in your digestive tract. Candida is a form of yeast, and it tells your brain to gorge yourself on sugar and other bad ingredients, so it can grow in your body. That can lead to obesity and diabetes, alcohol dependency, and produce fungal and yeast infections throughout your body. If you have dandruff and your scalp itches, you have it.

There are other non-prescription options that are helpful you can find online that work to diminish sugar cravings, usually under candida or yeast headings. I had to eliminate sugar, including high fructose corn syrup from my diet, and continue to use health food store candida fighters. I don't think I would have been able to conquer cancer as long as I was feeding it what it wants. The best suggestion I have for you is to read labels on food. Sugar is added to nearly every processed grocery item in the supermarket. Going organic and sticking to unprocessed food may be your best bet to avoid excess sugar in your diet. When you can look at pastries and cakes on display in your store's bakery aisle and walk on by without feeling a twinge of desire, congratulations, you've made it.

My personal story of surviving cancer involves mostly natural and nonmedical means. When the cancer first attacked my spine and my hip, I could barely sleep, walk, or focus on anything else. I was in terrible pain. I was shocked to learn that cancer had spread to my bones and possibly my kidney and liver. In 2015, nearly two years after the two lumpectomies, I had multiple areas of my body invaded with this disease. Because I had been given the all clear after my lumpectomy, I was puzzled why it had spread. I theorized that because I had to have two lumpectomies within a two week period, it had spread during that time. If the hospital had had an onsite lab that could verify clear margins in the tissue removed from my breast, perhaps it might not have. I did not even take that into consideration when choosing a hospital for this procedure, although I vaguely recall they may have mentioned that to me beforehand. If you are ever in this situation, it may be a good thing to consider before choosing your hospital. Most likely, because I didn't make any dietary changes or add anticancer supplements, the small amount of cancer cells left behind were given a license to grow in my body unopposed.

Chapter 8:
Toss Your Junk and
Get the Lead Out

On one occasion early after my hip surgery, I spoke with an overweight older lady I had never met before at a church luncheon. She was newly diagnosed with breast cancer. She was nearly crying as she shared her fears with everyone at the table over her cherry pie and ice cream. As we were leaving, I walked out with her, and told her in private about my conversation with the technician regarding the sugar and cancer link, and she could not get away from me fast enough. She abruptly ended the conversation, because apparently all she wanted was sympathy, and not helpful information. It's a choice people have to make. She chose to keep eating junk food and desserts like pies and cakes, and a month later I saw her again dining on heaping amounts of sweets. Choosing to live requires us to do everything in our power to change the lifestyle that may have contributed to cancer. Some people just aren't willing to make that sacrifice. Those sweet desserts may just cost you an arm or a leg, or a breast, and maybe eventually your life.

Dr. Seyfried writes in his book "Cancer as a

Metabolic Disease" that "Protection of mitochondria from oxidative damage will prevent or reduce risk of cancer". In other words, antioxidants like Vitamins A, C, D, and E, Omega 3 fatty acids, and minerals such as selenium and magnesium can combat free radicals that can lead to cancer. Oxidative damage is caused by free radicals, which are often caused by exposure to radiation and toxic substances in our food and environment. Some studies used by the National Cancer Institute to refute the value of antioxidants in preventing cancer used very low levels of vitamins and minerals in those studies. I have always used larger amounts of them, especially since facing a deadly disease so they are more effective. Selenium is critical for life according to the January/February 2017 issue of Life Extension magazine. The article "Selenium's Impact on Cancer Reduction" indicates that low selenium in the body raises the risk for colorectal cancer, liver cancer, and prostate cancer. One study in 1996 showed that "200 mcg of selenium daily was associated with a 50% reduction in the risk of dying from cancer". Optimal selenium levels provide protection against all types of cancer according to the article, including cervical cancer. Selenium is a trace element that lowers fasting blood sugar, insulin and insulin resistance, all factors associated with increased cancer risk.

From Dr. Seyfried's book and other sources, I learned that diet is very important to recovery. Not just what to avoid, but what to add. I believe the junk food that we put into our bodies, like nitrates and nitrites in lunchmeat, ham and hotdogs are harmful chemicals that may be responsible for cancer growth. I eliminated these and other processed food and diet sodas and anything with high fructose corn syrup. Fresh and frozen vegetables, salads topped with a small dash of vinegar and fresh olive oil, unprocessed chicken and fish, and some fruits were the bulk of my diet. I learned to never use old or rancid olive oil or any other cooking oil that's been sitting for a long time. There is some controversy about what kind of oil is best for cooking, but in my research, canola oil didn't rank too high. Fresh fruit goes well with plain yogurt and is good for your digestive health. I lost over 50 pounds, which also relieved pressure on my artificial hip.

I still maintain a healthy weight of 120 pounds. Of course, a bland diet can discourage people very quickly into thinking that a little cheating won't hurt, or maybe all this sacrifice won't really help at all. At times, I found myself thinking that it's ridiculous for me to believe that changing my diet and taking supplements could really heal me when the entire medical conglomeration says they have the only effective cancer treatments. Even though I had no reassurance from anybody else that it would work, I kept following this food and supplement regimen because for me the alternative was literally death.

I switched to a variety of sweeteners like Stevia, honey, and monk fruit that don't cause sugar cravings. The taste takes some getting used to, but it's worth it. I found that apples, grapes and blueberries are fine to snack on, and I added broccoli, cauliflower, spinach, carrots, tomatoes, kale, and fish to my diet. I rarely eat pork or beef. I drink juices like orange, grapefruit, pineapple, cranberry, pomegranate, and grape. I avoid fruit drinks that are mostly high fructose corn syrup, and instead drink 100% juice. I mix pineapple and grapefruit juice together for breakfast, or orange and grapefruit juice. Green tea is also a good choice for a beverage. I have eliminated wine and other alcohol. Alcohol and cigarettes together cause higher incidences of lung, mouth and throat cancers than cigarettes or alcohol alone. People generally die quickly from these cancers, so once you have a diagnosis of oral or throat cancer, it's hard to beat.

Beyond the sugar restrictions, and other changes in my diet, I knew there had to be more things I needed to do to keep living. I picked up magazines, scoured the internet, and read library books on cancer. I read many helpful articles claiming ways to lower your chances of getting cancer. I found an online article called "New Study finds that Spirulina can Help Treat Pancreatic Cancer" originally published in the March-April 2014 issue of the Annals of Hepatology. Researchers used mice and humans as test subjects and found that spirulina can stimulate antibodies, improve white blood cell count, and decrease proliferation of pancreatic cancer cells in all test subjects versus a control group. Spirulina is basically a freshwater algae packed with nutrients. It is available in health food stores and it is a part of my supplement regimen. A few articles also offered information on reducing cancer if you already have it. I am grateful I had the power to find information that allowed me to choose a different approach than is espoused by the medical profession, because I succeeded in eliminating my cancer.

Also, please check food labels and take the time to look up ingredients. The junk that we put into our bodies that contain harmful chemicals are cited in numerous publications as potential causes of cancer. A hundred years ago, cancer was very rare. I believe it's no coincidence that cancer has exploded as our food has been fertilized with cancer causing chemicals and modified to include more and more harmful chemicals and added sugars. We are also being exposed to chemicals that kill weeds and pollute our air and water at an alarming rate.

Chapter 9:
It's Never Too Late

When I started researching non-medical cures for cancer, I was already at Stage IV breast cancer. For a cancer patient, that's the worst diagnosis you can get. It's an automatic terminal disease diagnosis. Six months the doctor gave me. Within two years of my initial Stage I diagnosis in 2013, I had gone from an excised lump in my left breast to a full out body invasion of cancer cells. I knew what the medical profession had to offer me. Besides the anti-estrogen pills, and prescription Ibrance, there was only radiation, chemotherapy, and surgery. The radiologist literally told me "that's all we have to offer you". What? After all the decades and millions of dollars given to medical research facilities and to the American Cancer Society, and that's it? What I had left to try was chemo, and that wasn't going to work for me. It was a non-starter. I would just increase my misery and shorten my life. It made me wonder how even fifteen to twenty percent of us terminally ill breast cancer survivors make it to the five-year mark.

Let me be clear that I am in favor of having cancerous tumors removed if your chances of surviving the surgery are good. It gives you a head start in your recovery. I benefitted greatly from surgery, which reduced a large portion of cancer cells, but not all of them. It's never a good idea to think the battle's over with the surgery. Cancer can travel through your lymph nodes or your bloodstream and, like a busy beaver, start building a dam of cancer cells anywhere it chooses. Treating it with chemo is like setting your hair on fire to fix a bad hair day. It can damage your heart, your intestines, your brain, your nervous system, and leave you in chronic pain. The list of potential damages is lengthy so before you do it, look it up and weigh the pros and cons.

For me, the protocol I used began to show progress within 4 to 5 weeks. The pain subsided and follow-up tests showed cancer cells shrinking. Today, I can walk, drive, do laundry, bend over, put on my socks, work out on the treadmill at the YMCA, go up and down steps, read, and write. Everything still works, and I haven't lost any limbs. I am not in any pain, unless I sit too long and then my artificial hip protests. A brain scan showed that cancer in my skull didn't invade my brain. I am grateful that I am not in pain anymore.

I have to contrast what I did for my cancer to the medical field's ongoing, never-ending research that gobbles up millions of dollars every year and puts out only a few positive results. They promise that a cure is only a few years away and your donation will help speed things up. Any new treatments are unaffordable for average people since most aren't covered by insurance, so wealthy clients are first served. For instance, President Jimmy Carter survived Melanoma, a type of skin cancer that had spread to his liver and brain. He was treated with surgery, radiation and a treatment that was approved for use by the U.S. Food and Drug Administration in 2014, according to a 2016 NBC news online article titled "Cancer Drug Keytruda Keeps Some Patients Alive for 3 Years". After receiving this treatment from August 2015 through February 2016, Carter was declared cancer- free in March 2016. The NBC article states that about fifteen percent of Keytruda patients obtain complete remission like Carter, while forty percent only live for an average of three years after treatment. The majority, about sixty percent die within two years. I refused chemo because I believe that your body's immune system will attack and kill cancer cells if allowed to do so. Keytruda research confirms that belief. Rather than destroy a patient's immune system like chemotherapy does, Keytruda works to bolster a patient's immune system so it can do its job of seeking out and destroying cancer cells. With Keytruda, the medical community has now developed treatments which include enhancing the body's own immune system to attack and kill cancer cells, primarily melanoma and lung cancer. They're looking in the right direction. Of course, they give no credit to natural immune boosters like Vitamin C, Echinacea and Goldenseal.

In 2015 my nephew died from the same cancer that President Carter was successfully treated for that same year. At the time, treatment with Keytruda cost about $12,500 a month, a sum he could not afford, and his insurance did not cover. Radiation and chemotherapy only made his suffering worse. My nephew took an expensive experimental medication, most likely Keytruda, that cost him $10,000 a month out of pocket, near the end of his life. He trusted his doctors who were affiliated with a prestigious hospital, but the treatments swere ineffective. He died soon after, a mere three weeks after my own Stage IV diagnosis, and before I could advise him of my research. He, like so many others, trusted his doctors and followed their advice without seeking his own cure using alternative solutions. They, of course, gouged him financially and in my opinion just let him die. Promising therapies from the medical profession won't help if you can't pay for them. Medical insurance companies don't like to cover experimental treatments and most of them don't work anyway. Average people just suffer and die, even after decades of research and millions of dollars spent. Bolstering my own immune system has been my mission since the metastasis occurred. It has never made any sense to me to have a chemical injected into my body that's guaranteed to destroy my immune system, like chemo does. Instead of helping the body's natural defenses, chemo destroys them, leaving patients susceptible to cancer's return and other opportunistic infections with a vengeance.

There are supplements that are believed to help the immune system fight off cancer cells. Echinacea is one of them. I had taken it occasionally after reading that it helps prevent the flu and the common cold. Since my hip surgery, I have taken 400 mg of Echinacea every day. I have not been ill with the flu or a cold since, and I believe it has helped keep my cancer from spreading. If I start to get the sniffles or a sore throat, I double my dose of Vitamin C and take it every hour until they're gone, usually within three hours. Some research I found seems to point to Vitamin C as a treatment for cancer and I take 1,000 mg daily. My cousin Kenny who died from lung cancer in 2016 was in remission after surgery and radiation and chemo, for about a year. Then it came back with a vengeance and killed him. Except for the grace of God, that would have been my fate.

It's very important to stop ingesting cancer-causing chemicals in food. If you have cancer, stop eating foods that make cancer explode throughout your body. Take supplements that don't harm you and may in fact reduce your cancer. I beat the odds after being diagnosed with metastatic breast cancer. The idea of dying was always in my thoughts during those first days. It was only when I was looking online and reading books and magazines that I was able to keep those morbid thoughts away. I never lost focus, and I believe that's why I persisted and kept looking for answers until I found them. Most cancer patients believe the doctors to the exclusion of all else. Their hope has been misplaced because it is based upon old and useless treatments that do not work for most, and in fact make their condition much, much worse. Why do doctors continue to offer us these treatments that only buy us a little more time? It may not be their fault. Maybe they haven't been informed during their medical training about other options. Maybe they've been taught to believe that natural remedies are bogus and prescription medications along with surgery, radiation, and chemotherapy and the newest experimental therapy are the only treatments to recommend. Or maybe the cancer industry is designed to keep us in the dark.

Chapter 10:
A Skin Cream that
Can Heal Cancer?

I have successfully prolonged my life well past my projected expiration date. What other incredible things have I done to halt cancer from progressing? The answer is so simple, so very simple that at times, even I can't believe it worked so well. It's this simple: Change your food, your water, avoid things that increase your risk (like cancer causing chemicals), and use an over the counter cream on your skin. One of my initial steps to recovery was an unusual one and something I had no reason to believe would work.

In June 2015, shortly after my release from the hospital after my hip surgery, I was given a topical cream by a family member who had done some research on cancer cures in an effort to save my life. He had an idea that it would work and recommended that I apply it on my skin over the areas where cancer was active in my body. I knew I had cancer in my spine, left femur, skull and possibly a kidney and my liver. So, I applied the cream over those areas, once a day after showering. Within three weeks, the pain in my spine subsided and the hip and upper femur pain also lessened. Within two months a bone scan showed cancer was retreating from my spine and by the next year, it was totally gone. I continue to use the cream to this day. As of 2016, my X-rays, CT scans, bone scans, and brain scans are all negative for cancer. I believe it worked to eliminate the cancer in my body, along with the other changes I made.

I shared my topical treatment with a male friend who survives to this day after a lung cancer diagnosis two years ago. He was told by three doctors, one local and two at a renowned cancer clinic, that they were 99% sure he had lung cancer in both lungs. A heavy smoker, he was in his late 50's when he got that news. He began applying the cream on his chest over his lungs daily for two months. He also had COPD and a biopsy was very risky for him due to the strong possibility of having a lung collapse "like a pierced balloon" they had told him.

On the day the biopsy and possible lung removal was scheduled at the clinic, they did another scan of his lungs and sent him home. He called me and excitedly told me they cancelled his surgery. When I asked why he replied, "They did a scan and it showed the masses have nearly disappeared, so they said it wasn't cancer after all, because cancer doesn't shrink". What? The doctors had never seen lung cancer cells shrink without surgical intervention. "Then what was it?" I asked him. He said they didn't know what else it could be, but because it was clearing up, it could not be cancer. So, the medical doctors didn't believe their own diagnosis because his tumors were shrinking. That was good news for him because it means the topical cream appears to work for other types of cancer beside breast cancer. Luckily, my friend avoided the pain and damage to his lungs from surgery and he is cancer free today. I believe it worked for him to eliminate his lung cancer and that bolsters my own belief that it helped eliminate my cancer also.

So, what is this "miracle" cream? Surprisingly, it's an over the counter, naturally sourced estriol cream that my brother recommended to me. He gave me a jar that he bought online. I mention naturally sourced because there are artificially sourced products and I don't believe they are effective. I recommend that you stay away from them. Natural estriol cream can be found online and there are several distributors. I won't endorse any one in particular. Because it was an estrogen, I was initially afraid to try it. My type of cancer was estrogen positive, meaning estrogen fueled its growth. My brother had to convince me to try it because of my fear of it making it worse. Then he tried the: "What have you got to lose?" approach. He was right. I was dying anyway.

His research into breast cancer came because I was diagnosed with it and given six months to live. I learned from him there are actually three types of estrogen: Estriol, Estrone, and Estradiol. He had found an article from an obscure 1966 study in the Journal of the American Medical Association (JAMA) that indicated natural estriol seemed to inhibit breast cancer in test mice and in women. The other two types, estrone and estradiol, may actually encourage cancer growth in breast tissue. I started to apply it on my skin shortly after my hip surgery anywhere I knew cancer resided inside my body and anywhere I had pain. Later, he sent me copies of the pages from the JAMA article titled "Reduced Estriol Excretion in Patients with Breast Cancer Prior to Endocrine Therapy" which starts on page 112 of Volume 196 and ends on page 120 of the JAMA Journal dated June 27, 1966. The study states "Unlike estrone and estradiol, which are carcinogenic for the mammary glands of rodents upon chronic administration to males or castrated females, estriol and its isomers have not thus far been shown to be carcinogenic." The study, conducted in Boston, involved women with breast cancer and a control group of non-cancerous women. One observation was that the breast cancer group excreted less estriol in their urine than the non-cancerous group, presumably because they had less estriol in their system. On page 118 of the journal, the author states that "Visceral breast carcinoma metastases have been reported to regress after therapy with estriol..." meaning breast cancer cells in soft tissue organs like lungs and kidneys showed regression after therapy with estriol. The study also found that "Likewise, objective remission of metastases has been noted after testosterone, cortisol or prednisone therapy in 20% to 30% of patients with metastases." I don't recall anyone on my medical team suggesting that any of these could help me. Isn't it odd that the study results have been apparently overlooked by everyone in the medical field for over fifty years?

Almost as interesting is the ability for the 1966 study authors to look into the future and speculate that the birth control pill would contribute to an increase in breast cancer. Here's what they said on the subject: "The declining birth rate in the U.S. and other countries, partly resulting from chronic hormonal therapy inhibiting ovulation, may lead to increased mammary cancer incidence in the future." At the time of the study, the birth control pill had just been approved six years prior, in 1960. I was twenty when I started using the pill and nearly thirty before I stopped. It's possible it may have been a factor in my own bout of breast cancer at age sixty one. Estriol is more abundant during pregnancy, where it provides support for the growing fetus. There is much more to the study, but the gold nugget is that estriol has been known by medical researchers to reduce metastatic breast cancer since I was fourteen years old. I find it extremely depressing to know that this information has been suppressed for all these years. In fact, I was deterred from using estrogen, and the different types, estriol, esterone, and estradiol were never differentiated in any of my medical reports, nor explained to me by my doctors.

At the time I started using it, we didn't know if it would work. To our knowledge, no one had ever tried it topically before. The research done fifty years ago was never reproduced that we could find.

So, I was the lab rat, so to speak. If it worked, I might survive. Fortunately, it did. And if it worked on breast cancer, it may just work on other types of cancer. I am personally aware that it works on skin cancer, specifically squamous and basal cell carcinoma. I had several small growths removed from my face, shoulders, arms and neck during the two years between my Stage I and Stage IV cancer diagnoses. I also had two growths develop on my shoulders shortly after my Stage IV diagnosis. For those two bumps, I used the natural estriol cream, just a small dab once daily on the growths. Within four weeks they were gone. They just shrunk away and have not returned. I have not had any other skin cancers develop since that time.

Estriol is available solo as a cream and is not very costly. It works well as a skin cream, because it is easy to apply, readily absorbed through skin, and takes only small amounts to be effective. It may work best when combined with a healthy lifestyle including vitamins and supplements and lifestyle changes. I have never relied on it alone to reduce my cancer, but I really believe it contributed the most to my recovery out of all the other changes I made. Since the first few weeks after my terminal diagnosis, I have used just a few dabs daily on my chest area, over my liver, my hip and femur, kidney area and spine. I still use it today along with the shotgun approach of vitamins, minerals and a healthy diet, not trusting any one thing to keep cancer away.

Interestingly, UCLA researchers are studying the use of estriol to treat people with Multiple Sclerosis (MS) to help regenerate the myelin sheath, the coating on nerve cells that's destroyed by the autoimmune disease. According to the article on the Daily Bruin online, "Estriol, a type of estrogen produced by the fetal placenta, was found to act specifically on the brain cells that produce myelin". A series of small clinical trials have delivered promising results. A larger study of 1,000 patients is being planned. If you have MS, and aren't part of this university study, this may be of interest to you. You can try it at home by using estriol cream on your skin. The researchers have evidence that estriol treats the cause of MS, not just the symptoms. For me, it caused my cancer pain to subside and after a few months, the scans and tests showed cancer to be disappearing from my body. Use only naturally sourced estriol.

One thing I want to say about being a cancer

victim is that it's a very traumatic experience. It helps to have positive people in your life. If you are dealing with stressful people, the less time you spend with them the better you will feel. I also spent plenty of time after my diagnosis looking backwards and blaming myself for getting cancer and for all the other bad decisions I had made. Looking backwards and blaming yourself is not helpful. But understanding what you did wrong and changing course is. Be kind to yourself. Take negative emotions out of it as much as you can. Your body is a machine and it takes certain substances to make it work properly. A few months ago, just as I was considering writing this book, I saw an online post from someone who was leaving town and selling everything she owned to move to a state that allowed assisted suicide. She had terminal cancer like me. How depressed and hopeless she must have felt to make such a sad decision. It's for people like her that I am sharing my story.

Chapter 11:
Vitamins and Minerals
to Take for Life

My research led me to consider a whole host of supplements, herbs and vitamins. Since research has shown that cancer patients are often Vitamin D deficient, and my initial tests showed that my levels were below recommended levels, I started taking 2000 to 4000 IU of Vitamin D3 daily. Vitamin D helps you fight off certain cancers. Vitamin D lowers your risk of developing colorectal and other cancers, but by itself does not prevent cancer. It's a good bullet to put in your cancer fighting arsenal. The next item I found that may be beneficial is curcumin found in the spice turmeric. It comes in a capsule and has been associated with cancer inhibition. If you Google it you will see many articles on its cancer fighting properties, notably on breast, colon, and skin cancers. There are many articles you can find on the internet about turmeric. One recent one by Dr. Timothy Moynihan, MD of the Mayo Clinic, says "Curcumin is thought to have antioxidant properties, which means it may decrease swelling and inflammation". Lab and animal research suggest that curcumin may prevent cancer, slow the spread of cancer, make chemotherapy more effective and protect healthy cells from damage by radiation therapy. Curcumin is being studied for use in many types of cancer. The article also says more research is needed, but why wait for that? I've been taking it for three years and believe it's a part of the reason I am still here.

I also read in the January/February 2015 edition of Life Extension Magazine that environmental factors may be responsible for up to ninety percent of cancers. The troublemakers are things we are exposed to daily, like plastic cups and containers, food packaging, cigarette smoke, pesticides, nitrites in our meats, aluminum in pots and deodorant, and loads of toady stuff in our tap water. Whatever else you do, STOP drinking unfiltered tap water. If you want to know why, just have it tested. Whether it's city or well water, you don't know what you're getting. You only need to look at Flint, Michigan's tap water scandal, which has poisoned thousands of children and adults with lead. Most city water pipes still have lead in them, which can end up in your body.

The article "Lead - American Cancer Society" on Cancer.org highlights a study that shows cancer in lab animals increased when they were exposed to lead from contaminated water. Kidney tumors have been linked to lead in people as have tumors in the brain, lung and other organs. Apparently, fluoride may be hazardous too, and it is in all city water everywhere and even in most toothpaste. My primary choice for hydration is sterilized or filtered water with lemon. Baking soda is an effective toothpaste substitute.

Another enormous concern is the fact that cancer-causing chemicals are routinely sprayed on our fruits and vegetables. It's impossible to protect against all carcinogens, (even our carpets have formaldehyde in them), so we need to neutralize them. One effective means to do that is taking chlorophyllin, derived from chlorophyll, which gives plants their green color. The Life Extension article claims "chlorophyllin may protect your body from cancer-causing agents and promote growth of healthy cells". This happens because it binds to mutated substances (carcinogens) and helps excrete them from the body.

One study they cite involves a fungal toxin

abundant in corn and soy sauce grown in China in a high-risk area for liver cancer. Individuals who took 100 mg of chlorophyllin three times a day for three months had a higher excretion rate of compounds associated with liver cancer risk. This means the chlorophyllin was binding to the carcinogens and excreting them from the body, dropping the risk of developing liver cancer. I figured if it works for liver cancer it won't hurt to try it with breast cancer. I found a supplement called Chlorella, which is an ingestible source of chlorophyll that's available online and in most vitamin stores. I take a 500 mg tablet every day.

Life Extension magazine also lists selenium as a mineral critical for life. In "Selenium's Impact on Cancer Reduction" in their January/February 2017 issue it cited research published in the Journal of the American Medical Association that showed people taking selenium supplements had a significant reduction in colorectal, lung, and prostate cancers, with a fifty percent reduction in the risk of mortality for all cancers." The test subjects were given 200 mcg of selenium daily during the study along with zinc, and vitamins A, C and E. The article also cited a study of women in 2015 with precancerous cervical lesions that subsided with selenium.

Cervical lesions are precursors to cervical cancer.

Magnesium is another mineral that is important in maintaining a healthy body. Magnesium has a role in balancing calcium. Calcium makes muscles contract. Magnesium allows muscles to relax. Excess calcium deposits end up in our arteries, becoming plaque, and leading to high blood pressure and heart attacks. Excess calcium in your joints causes chronic pain, arthritis, muscle or nerve pain. Magnesium dissolves excess calcium, allowing muscles and arteries to relax and reducing high blood pressure since this muscle-relaxing effect also applies to the heart and arteries.

But here is the cancer connection. Our DNA contains instructions on how new cells should subdivide and grow. When magnesium levels are too low, the cell walls weaken, and newly formed cells can be incomplete or changed to create abnormal cell growth. New cells take instructions from the altered DNA and multiply with those instructions causing cellular mutations. According to the online article "Magnesium Deficiency and Cancer" this is the beginning of cancer since cancer is abnormal cell growth. Their conclusion is that magnesium deficiency can lead to the start of cancer as well as hinder treatment. I included magnesium supplementation to my regimen early on after reviewing several similar articles about it.

The Standard American Diet (SAD) is often lacking in the best food sources for magnesium which are green leafy vegetables, fruits, fish, nuts, and legumes. Further damage to our soil from the use of pesticides, herbicides and fertilizers have diminished magnesium in our soil so plants no longer have much of the mineral to absorb from the ground. The US daily recommended amount of magnesium is 300 to 400 mg of magnesium daily. If your diet is very SAD, consisting of sugary, processed, fatty junk and fast food, you likely need supplementation. Small positive changes in your diet over time will reduce your risk of chronic diseases including cancer. I also added black cumin seed oil to my diet after reading that it may help fight cancer and have tumor reducing properties. I believe it helped with my weight loss.

I received my Stage IV Breast Cancer diagnosis on May 29, 2015, and it's been six years since my initial breast cancer diagnosis in 2013. My prosthetic hip works well. Multiple tests have confirmed that I am cancer free and have been since early in 2016. In April of 2016, a year after my Stage IV diagnosis, and several months after I discontinued Letrozole, a bone scan found that the increased activity which indicates active cancer cells in my spine and skull and femur had diminished, and I no longer had signs of cancer in those or any other locations. X-rays of my left hip prosthesis show it in remarkably good condition. The surrounding leg bone (femur) that holds it in place is no longer cancerous. I do not have osteoporosis. If the cancer had continued to destroy my femur, the prosthesis would not be able to support my leg. Yet for four years it has maintained its integrity. I cannot predict the future and cannot say with certainty that my breast cancer won't come back, but I feel as long as I keep doing the things I have been doing, I stand a better than average chance that it won't.

I know it's hard to know what to do when you are facing cancer. After my first bout of breast cancer, I did nothing different, and it came back and nearly killed me. For me, a mix of medical care, including surgery, some radiation, and the short term use of an anti-hormone drug helped buy me some time. If medical interventions alone had been responsible for the reversal of metastatic cancer in my body, I would be delighted to say so. I will say the surgeries helped me tremendously. Having the lumpectomies and the hip replacement surgeries definitely extended my life. After that, I was literally dying to try something else, so I relied on a change of diet, supplements, and estriol cream to help eliminate cancer from my body. I have included some excerpts from my medical records below showing that I went from active Stage I to Stage IV breast cancer and then to cancer-free.

The first page of the pathology report below dated September 20, 2013 is the biopsy report I got before my first lumpectomy on November 1, 2013. It shows a left breast mass. The next page is the pathology report that was done in May 2015. It shows a diagnosis of metastatic breast cancer in my left femur, just below where my left hip bone was removed and replaced with titanium. A lytic lesion is an area of weakened bone, and can be a hole in the bone, caused by cancer. The ER positive means it is Estrogen Responsive breast cancer, meaning estrogen makes it grow.

```
PATIENT: THOMAS,                    ACCT #: H02069824247 LOC:  H.US       U #: H000155769
                                    AGE/SX: 61/F         ROOM:            REG: 09/17/13
REG DR:        Gregory M            DOB:    04/20/52     BHD:             DIS:
                                    STATUS: REG CLI      TLOC:
```

Specimen: **S-7753-13**

```
                    Spec Type: SURG            Ord. Dr.:       Gregory M
                    Status: SOUT               Collect Date:   09/17/13 1001
                                               Received Date:  09/17/13 1207
```

Source: A   Breast, NOS(LEFT BREAST MASS)
Procedure: GROSS AND MICRO, PR, CERB-2, CONTROL,RABBIT, ER, BREAST, NEEDLE,
                E-CADHERIN, P63, CONTROL, MOUSE, H&E/2, UNSTAINED SL/4, P120

PRE-OP DIAGNOSIS: LEFT BREAST MASS
POST-OP DIAGNOSIS: NONE GIVEN
SURGICAL PROCEDURE: LEFT BREAST CORE BIOPSY

DIAGNOSIS

A.   Left breast mass, core biopsy:
     INFILTRATING DUCTAL CARCINOMA, MODERATELY DIFFERENTIATED

COMMENT

Immunohistochemical stains were done on section A1 with the following results:
     ER: Positive (+3, 95%)
     PR: Negative (less than 1%)
     HER-2/neu: Equivocal (+2)
     E-cadherin: Positive in tumor cells, confirming their ductal origin.
     P120: Positive membrane staining in tumor cells, confirming their ductal origin.
     p63: Negative in tumor cells, supporting the diagnosis.

104

Orderable Name   Ordering Provider   Collected Date/Time
5/27/2015 07:35 EDT

Procedure   Result
Surgical   SEE BELOW(c) (R)

Corrected Results
c1:   Surgical
     Result comment modified on 6/16/2015 16:19 EDT by Contributor_system, SOFTLAB

     NAME: THOMAS,   ACCESSION NO: 15-SU-6491

       COPIES TO: PATH REPORTS MSO ;

     DIAGNOSIS:
     RIGHT FEMORAL HEAD:
     - METASTATIC POORLY DIFFERENTIATED CARCINOMA COMPATIBLE WITH BREAST
     ORIGIN.

       ER: MODERATELY STRONGLY POSITIVE IN GREATER THAN 90% OF TUMOR CELL
     NUCLEI.
     PR: NEGATIVE (0)
     HER2neu: NEGATIVE (1+)

     PROCEDURE: LEFT TOTAL HIP ARTHROPLASTY
     PRE-OP DX: LYTIC LESION LEFT FEMUR
     POST-OP DX: SAME

     SPECIMEN: FEMORAL HEAD, LEFT

     GROSS DESCRIPTION:
     Received labeled: Thomas,

     Received in formalin labeled "left femoral head" is a 4.2 x 4.1 x 3.3
     cm femoral head with up to 2 cm of attached neck. There is a small
     amount of adherent soft tissue between the head and the neck. The
     surgical margin is tan-red and straight. The articular surface is
     tan-red and smooth to slightly rough. The margin is inked and sectioned
     to show a 2 cm in greatest dimension rubbery/firm pale-tan well to
     ill-defined lesion that extends to the surgical margin. The remaining

LAB LEGEND: (c) = Corrected Result   A = Abnormal   C = Critical   H = High   L = Low

Report Request ID: 22986902   Page 11 of 13   Print Date/Time: 8/29/2015 15:27 EDT

The next image below lists the results of a full body bone scan taken June 4, 2015 while I was in the hospital following hip replacement surgery. They found a small area of increased activity in the left T10 transverse process. The T10 refers to a vertebra in the spinal column, and this "increased activity" was not seen on the prior study on November 22, 2013. The report also acknowledged an osteolytic lesion that showed up on the CT scan of the Left T10 vertebra taken the day before on June 3, 2015. To interpret, increased activity means cells are dividing rapidly, an indicator for cancer. It can also mean cells are being replaced following surgery. An osteolytic lesion is an area of softened bone that shows up as a hole on an X-ray or scan due to decreased bone density caused by cancer.

Osteolytic lesions appear in bone with breast cancer. Lesions in the spine like I had can lead to pain because of pressing down of nerves in the spinal cord (compression) and carry a risk of bone fracture. CT scans can show if a cancer has spread to the bone. When it has, your cancer has metastasized. This report also incorporates the results of the CT head scan of June 3, 2015 which shows a subtle osteolytic lesion in the left frontal calvarium (skull) consistent with a metastasis. So on June 3rd and again on June 4th, 2015, shortly after my hip surgery for metastatic breast cancer, I was diagnosed with Stage IV breast cancer because in addition to my hip and femur, I had breast cancer cells in in my spine and a lytic lesion consistent with cancer in my skull. According to the online article "Bone Metastasis Treatment with Medications" bone metastases is a result of cancer and "Bone metastases means your cancer is advanced and not curable".

EXAM DATE/TIME	PROCEDURE	ORDERING PROVIDER	STATUS
6/4/2015 13:10 EDT	NM Bone Imaging Whole Body	SCHNEIDER MD.,PHILIP A.	Auth (Verified)

NM Bone Imaging Whole Body

ORIGINAL

NM BONE IMAGING WHOLE BODY
Total Body Bone Scan

Clinical Statement: Bone mets . Breast carcinoma.

Comparison: Bone scan 11/22/2013, CT head, CT chest abdomen pelvis 6/3/2015

Technique:
Radiopharmaceutical: Tc 99m Methylene Diphosphonate IV Dose: 34.5 mCi
Anterior and posterior whole body images
Anterior and Posterior oblique views of the pelvis

Report: There has been interval placement of a LEFT total hip prosthesis. There is moderate activity diffusely surrounding the prosthesis consistent with the recent surgery (5/27/2015). There is a small site of increased activity in the LEFT T10 transverse process which is new since the prior study. On review of the CT chest 6/3/2015, there is a subtle osteolytic lesion at this site, consistent with a metastasis. There is a subtle focus of increased activity in the LEFT frontal calvarium which is unchanged. On CT head 6/3/15 there is a subtle osteolytic lesion in the LEFT frontal calvarium consistent with a metastasis. Sites of probable degenerative uptake in the acromioclavicular joints and bilateral feet also noted.

IMPRESSION: Suspect metastatic lesions in the LEFT frontal calvarium and LEFT T10 transverse process.

108

RAD - Nuclear Medicine

EXAM DATE/TIME	PROCEDURE	ORDERING PROVIDER	STATUS
8/25/2015 15:44 EDT	NM Bone Imaging Whole Body		Auth (Verified)

NM Bone Imaging Whole Body

ORIGINAL

NM BONE IMAGING WHOLE BODY
Total Body Bone Scan

Clinical Statement: BREAST CA, OBS FOR MALIGNANCY

Comparison: Bone scan 06/04/2015, CT chest abdomen pelvis 08/24/2015, CT head, chest, abdomen and pelvis 06/30/2015

Technique:
Radiopharmaceutical: Tc 99m Methylene Diphosphonate IV Dose: 30.5 mCi
Anterior and posterior whole body images
Anterior and Posterior oblique views of the pelvis

Report: Very subtle increased activity is noted within the LEFT frontal calvarium. This is not significantly changed from the prior study. Slightly increased activity in the LEFT T10 transverse process is noted with interval improvement. The recent CT 08/24/2015 shows development of sclerosis at the LEFT T10 transverse process at the site previously demonstrating a small osteolytic lesion on the CT of 06/30/2015. This is likely a healing metastasis. No new lesions are identified. Evidence of a LEFT hip prosthesis is seen. Increased activity surrounding the prosthesis has diminished compared to the prior study. The intensity of activity surrounding a prosthesis is within the expected range considering recent placement of the prosthesis 05/27/2015. Scattered areas of peripheral joint activity typical for degenerative changes are stable compared to the prior study.

IMPRESSION: Mild activity at the LEFT T10 transverse process has improved from the prior study. Mild LEFT frontal calvarial uptake is similar to the prior study. No new lesions.

Interpreted By: t ,Marshall MD
Preliminary Report By: .: ,Marshall MD
Electronically Signed By. .   ,Marshall MD

LAB LEGEND:	(c) = Corrected Result	A = Abnormal	C = Critical	H = High	L = Low

The bone scan below was done on December 16, 2016, a year and a half after my hip surgery. When compared to the bone scan done August 25, 2015 (included above), you notice there is no mention of the Left T10 vertebra. In 2015, that vertebra was mentioned as a "healing metastasis". A year and a half later, long after I stopped the Letrozole, there is no activity in that area of my spine, meaning it is completely healed. The small focus of activity near the tip of the prostheses in my hip has gradually decreased over time.

This was explained to me to mean that the bone was healing, and "activity" indicates the formation of new mature bone than can take several years to form. The impression tells it all. "No new abnormality" in my bones. No change in the skull lesion either. It is unclear if that area was ever cancerous. A brain scan earlier showed no cancer in my brain. A mammogram on the same day as the bone scan below shows no evidence of malignancy. Sometimes breast cancer returns to the other breast. It did not come back there or anywhere else in my chest area.

EXAM DATE/TIME	PROCEDURE	ORDERING PROVIDER	STATUS
12/16/2016 12:49 EST	NM Bone Imaging Whole Body		Auth (Verified)

NM Bone Imaging Whole Body

ORIGINAL

NM BONE IMAGING WHOLE BODY
Total Body Bone Scan

Clinical Statement: BREAST CA, OBS

Comparison: 4/22/2016

Technique:
Radiopharmaceutical: Tc 99m Methylene Diphosphonate IV Dose: 30 mCi
Anterior and posterior whole body images
Anterior and Posterior oblique views of the pelvis

Report: There is a photopenic area representing the patient's left hip prosthesis. There is a small focus of activity near the tip of the prosthesis which has shown a gradual decrease when compared to multiple prior studies. Most likely this is residual postoperative uptake. There are several small site of degenerative uptake in the knees and in the acromioclavicular joints similar to the prior study. There is minimal activity in the left frontal calvarium which is similar to the prior study. No other abnormality is noted.

IMPRESSION: Subtle left frontal calvarial lesion is unchanged. No new abnormality. Degenerative changes.

EXAM DATE/TIME	PROCEDURE	ORDERING PROVIDER	STATUS
12/16/2016 13:35 EST	MA Mammo Screening Bilateral w/Tomo		Auth (Verified)

MA Mammo Screening Bilateral w/Tomo
There is no mammographic evidence of malignancy. A follow-up mammogram in 12 months is recommended. I have personally reviewed the images of the examination and agree with the findings and interpretation.

The physician's note below dated November 19, 2015, shows the diagnosis of Stage IV Terminal Bone Cancer of Breast Origin which was assigned in June of 2015. My doctor also noted that I had started taking the Letrozole intermittently. I didn't tell her I had actually quit using it. Letrozole only works to inhibit estrogen while you are taking it, and I had actually stopped taking it by this time, due to some unpleasant side effects like hair thinning. I want to mention that I am not advocating that anyone else stop taking any prescribed medication for cancer treatment. Your cancer treatment protocol is between you and your doctor. I am only recounting what I did and that I suffered no ill effects from stopping the Letrozole after I had implemented the alternatives I've outlined in these chapters.

6/22/15
I have revd her prev visit notes pmh etc and updated and noted as below
since her last visit she had left hip sirgery dr johnson for mets disease
she had path positive for poorly diff ductal ca cw breast cancer
er 50% pr neg and her2neu neg
she has not started rt or pt eyt
she has declined hormonal therapy
ctcap neg for systemic disease
bone scasn uptake left hip spine and skull
she doesnt want chemo
ps 1-2 using cane
11/19/15
I have revd her prev visit notes prnh etc and updated and noted as below
since her last viist she has been taking the letrozole states not taking dialy and was reminded
she received 10 out of the15 pall radiation treatments left hip and is ambulatory
SHE HAS PERSISTENT LEFT HIP PAIN AND IS CONSIDERING QUITTING HER JOB
SHE DOES HAVE STAGE 4 TERMINAL BONE CANCER OF BREAST ORIGIN
SHE HAS HYPERCALCEMIA TODAY
hair thinning is better
us thyroid showed goiter TSH T3T4 WERE ORDERED
interval restagng ctcap and bone scan 8/15 indicate t10 lesion with sclerosis , calvarial lesion
and left hip lesions, also thyroid densities and thyroid us suggested
she would like to re xgeva today tol well previously no dental issues reported and she does
see a dentist reg

Chapter 12:
Life Goes On

Today, my survival is something that I can take for granted. Most people think I should feel the opposite, that I shouldn't take life for granted. To me, it's no big deal anymore. And that's exactly where I want to be; alive and not obsessing about having cancer return. As long as I am vigilant and don't fall back to bad habits, like eating sugar or skipping my anti-cancer supplement regimen daily, I feel my life expectancy has returned to normal. I'm hopeful that more people with cancer will live longer and healthier. It's very upsetting to hear of friends or relatives who have died after taking chemo. I always wish they could have been helped before it was too late.

Eventually the medical community may "find" a cure for my type of cancer. It hasn't so far, and I am not waiting for them to catch up. They are way too far behind. For example, I watched a commercial recently on TV from a cancer hospital that made me cringe. In the ad, a woman, either a real doctor or an actor posing as one, was talking about a man who appeared in the commercial with her and said he had Lymphoma. She said his cancer medical team recommended chemotherapy and then stem cell therapy, "and when his cancer progressed", they considered him a candidate for a new therapy to unleash his immune system. I had to rewind it to hear it again. What she admitted to on national TV was that chemotherapy didn't work, then stem cell didn't work, then and only then, were they going to consider bolstering his immune system that they had literally destroyed with chemotherapy. Chemo does destroy your immune system, along with just about everything else in your body. How can you fight off cancer, other infections or illnesses with no immune system? You would think that attempts to bolstering or "unleashing" as she called it, his immune system should have been the first thing they did. This ad is currently running on a major network. Apparently, this is a breakthrough in cancer treatment.

The medical industry seems to need to spend years and millions of dollars on everything they do before it's available to the public. By contrast, everything I have been using to control my cancer can be found now online or in stores, and they don't require a second mortgage to buy them.

Do yourself a favor. If you want to live you

have to make healthy choices. Only after facing death within six months did I consider diet to be a factor. Bolster your immune system on your own before taking any poison that will kill it. Take Echinacea and Goldenseal. Eat your vegetables, fresh or frozen preferably. Quit sugaring. There are medications available that inhibit the overwhelming craving for sugar you may have. Your doctor knows about them. Your doctor can prescribe an anti-fungal medication that will help. You can find over-the- counter products at any vitamin store for yeast and candida overgrowth. If you have sugar or alcohol cravings, dandruff, short term memory loss, or yeast infections, you may need help to overcome them. Stevia, honey, monk fruit are substitutes I use that have not caused sugar cravings. Avoid high fructose corn syrup and processed meats containing nitrates and nitrites. After being told by a medical technician that sugar increases cancer, I stopped eating anything with real sugar in it, as much as possible. It's worth giving your body the nutrition it deserves. Taking the estriol cream and applying it topically to my body daily has contributed to my healing. I would recommend that option before trying chemo. Since chemo has a long-term survival rate of about three percent, it may not make much of a difference to your survival. In fact, many of the people receiving chemo are getting it as a palliative measure; just something to make the dying patient feel like their medical team is doing something, when it's really only helping your doctor pay for his vacation home in Florida.

I have reason to believe that diet changes and supplements will work best to improve health in a body that has not been ravaged by chemo. If you do decide to take chemo, it will help to have a stronger body with a healthier immune system first. Chemo can bring life-long side effects, like nerve damage, memory loss, osteoporosis and heart damage just to name a few. The choice is always up to the individual. If anything, I hope I have encouraged you to do more research on your particular type of cancer.

I am pleased to find that there is finally an acknowledgement from researchers that a bad diet does contribute to cancer. A recent study by Tufts University states that there is convincing evidence that a poor diet can lead to a twenty-five to thirty-eight percent increase in some cancers. Specifically, diets high in red and processed meats contribute to stomach and colorectal cancers and low fruit and vegetable consumption adds to mouth and throat cancer risks. Sugar sweetened drinks were also included as risk factors for these and breast and liver cancers as well. I believe that someday cancer will be easily prevented as well as cured and the world will look back at the current medical treatment with disbelief. Always remember your health and life is your responsibility to protect. No one will care more about your life than you will. For your sake and for the people who love and depend on you, please consider your treatment options wisely.

References

Henry, Derek. "Cancer Develops from Fungal Infections Like Candida". Naturalnews.com 1/20/2015

Batts, Vicki. "Cancer Researchers Don't Want a 'Cure', They Would Lose Billions". Newstarget.com 8/23/2016

"Higher Vitamin D levels may be linked to lower risk of cancer". WWW.BMJ.com

Wells, S.D., "Health Basics: The true history of cancer in the USA" www.naturalnews.com 12/30/2018

"Breast Cancer Hormone Receptor Status" www.cancer.org Last revised 9/25/2017.

Szabo, Liz, Kaiser Health News. "Dozens of New Cancer Drugs do Little to Improve Survival". USAToday.com 2/13/2017

Mouridsen, H. "Letrozole in advanced breast cancer: the PO25 trial" www.ncbi.nlm.nih.gov 2/27/2007

"Higher Vitamin D levels may be linked to Lower Risk of Cancer" www.bmj.com/company/newsroom/higher-vitamin-d-levels-may-be-linked-to-lower-risk-of-cancer

Fox, Maggie "Cancer Drug Keytruda Keeps Some Patients Alive For 3 Years." Nbcnews.com 5/18/16.

Seyfried, Thomas, PhD. "Cancer as a Metabolic

Disease" 2012. John Wiley & Sons, Hoboken NJ,

"Antioxidants and Cancer Prevention – National Cancer Institute" www.cancer.gov/ Reviewed 2/6/2017

Moynihan, Timothy, MD. "Curcumin: Can it slow cancer growth?" www.mayoclinic.org 11/3/2018

Battaglia, Gina, "Protect Yourself from Environmental Cancer" Life Extension Magazine Jan/Feb 2015.

"The Budwig diet". www.budwigcenter.com

Chadwick, Dara. "Can a Low-Acid Diet Help Prevent Cancer?" www.curetoday.com 8/18/ 2015

Thomas, John P. "The Cancer Industry is too Prosperous to Allow a Cure". Healthimpact news.com 8/15/2014

Coldwell, Leonard, MD. "Chemo and Radiation Treatment Does Not Work 97% of the Time." Youtube 8/9/2014

"Lead-AmericanCancerSociety".Cancer.org 5/27/2014

Greenwald, Julia. "Magnesium Deficiency and Cancer". Beat cancer.org July 12, 2015

Maltzman,Julia, MD."Bone Metastasis Treatment with Medications". www.oncolink.org/cancers/10/15/2018

Laino, Charlene."Low Vitamin D levels linked to Advanced Cancers" webmd.com/cancer/news 10/4/11
Mercola, J., MD "Is Vitamin D the New Silver Bullet for Cancer" articles/mercola.com 2/ 11/10

Mercola, J. MD "Laetrile Cancer Research Cover-up" https://articles.mercola.com. 10/18/2014

Ravensthorpe, Michael. "New Study finds that Spirulina can Help Treat Pancreatic Cancer". https://Healing the Body.Ca/

Lemon, Henry et.al. "Reduced Estriol Excretion in Patients with Breast Cancer Prior to Endocrine Therapy". JAMA Vol. 196 No. 13. 6/27/1966

Hill, Kennedy. "UCLA Researchers Work to Advance Tx targeting source of MS. theDailybruin.com 5/15/2019

Tufts University, Health Sciences Campus. "New Study Estimates Preventable Cancer Burden linked to Poor Diet in the U.S." www. sciencedaily.com. 5/22/2019

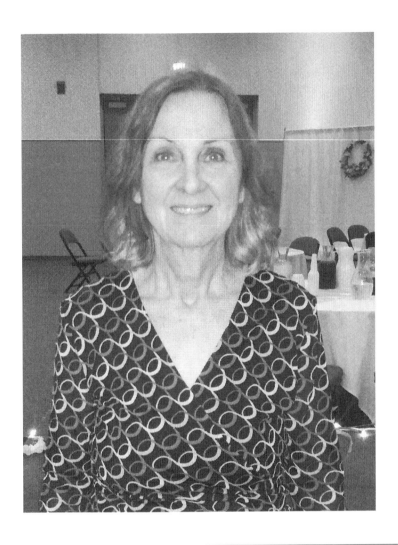

RENEE THOMAS is a retired Social Worker and first-time author. *Cancer-Free Naturally* is a journal of her struggle with Metastatic Breast Cancer. Ms. Thomas hopes her research and experience can also help others dealing with cancer. Ms. Thomas lives in Ohio with her youngest son and three cats.

Made in the
USA
Lexington, KY